PATIENTS BUILD YOUR PRACTICE

DISCLAIMER

This book is intended to help simplify the concepts and strategies of medical practice marketing. All information contained in this guide is based on the experience of the author and the recommendations are to be considered the opinion of the author. Neither the author nor the publisher may be held liable for any misuse or misinterpretation of the guidelines in this text. All information provided is believed and intended to be reliable, but accuracy cannot be guaranteed by the author or the publisher.

PATIENTS BUILD YOUR PRACTICE

WORD-OF-MOUTH MARKETING FOR HEALTHCARE PRACTITIONERS

Michael E. Cafferky

McGraw-Hill, Inc.
New York St. Louis San Francisco Auckland Bogatá Caracas
Lisbon London Madrid Mexico Milan Montreal New Delhi Paris
San Juan Singapore Sydney Tokyo Toronto

Patients Build Your Practice: Word-of-Mouth Marketing For Healthcare Practitioners

1 2 3 4 5 6 7 8 9 0 DOC DOC 954

ISBN 0-07-600676-X

This book was composed and set in Souvenir Light by Huron Valley Graphics, Inc.

TABLE OF CONTENTS

Preface xi

Chapter 1: Reality As We Know It 1

Negative Word-of-Mouth Happens More Than You Think 2

Perception Is Reality 4

The Positive Side of Word-of-Mouth 5

What They Are Talking About 7

Practical Suggestions In This Book 9

Chapter 2: What It Takes To Succeed In Word-of-Mouth Marketing 13

The Threshold of Excellent Service 13

Finding The Threshold 14

Other Success Factors 16

Chapter 3: Word-of-Mouth Marketing Theory 20

How Leaders Create Success For You 22

New Patients Use Opinion Leaders To Make Decisions 23

Why Would An Opinion Leader Talk About You? 25

Why Do Followers Listen? 25

When Does Your Reputation Spread? 26

Summary 27

Practical Ideas To Implement The Theory 28

Chapter 4: Patient Power With Clusters of People 35

What Are The Primary Word-of-Mouth Clusters? 36

Conclusion 54

Chapter 5: Stopping Negative Word-of-Mouth 55

Are Complainers Allies or Pests? 55

Avoid Isolation 57

Implement A Complaint-Gathering Program 57

Establish An "Instant Solution" Program 60

Heading Off Problems Before They Begin 63

Make Changes Visible and Communicate 65

Chapter 6: The Cost of Word-of-Mouth 67
Return on Investment 70
The Costs of Negative Word-of-Mouth 71
Chapter 7: Train, Train, Train 77
Sixteen Home-Grown Training Ideas 79
Chapter 8: Making Patients Into Champions: Ninety-Plus Things That Can Go Right (or Wrong) 86
Before The First Contact With The Doctor 86
Calling For An Appointment 87
Getting To The Office 88
Registration Process 88
Medical Service 90
Making Financial Arrangements 90
Leaving The Office 91
Follow-Up To The Visit 91
Chapter 9: Word-of-Mouth Marketing In Managed Care Settings 93
Why Use Word-of-Mouth In Managed Care? 94
Why Managed Care? 95
Sources of Satisfaction and Dissatisfaction 96
Challenges For Word-of-Mouth Marketing 97
Tactics For Solo Practitioners and Small Groups 98
Tactics For HMOs, IPAs, and Medical Groups 100
Chapter 10: Breaking Through Cultural Barriers With Word-of-Mouth Marketing 105
Culture's Power 106
Culture Is Learned Behavior 107
Common Values Build Your Reputation 108
What To Watch For 108
Identifying The Opinion Leaders 109
Chapter 11: Word-of-Mouth Marketing For Other Specific Groups 115
How To Pick A Community Group 117
Working With A Variety of Groups 118
How To Identify Patients' Involvement In Groups 124
How To Network In Social Groups 125
Conclusion 127

Chapter 12: Conclusion   128
Appendix 1: Sample Letters and Forms   133
Thank You For Your Referral Letter   134
Welcome To Our Practice Letter   135
Hall of Fame Introduction Letter   136
Welcome To A New Health Plan Member Letter   137
Appendix 2: Coordinating Word-of-Mouth With Other
Promotional Methods   138
Other Promotional Methods To Support Word-of-Mouth
Marketing   141
Appendix 3: Word-of-Mouth Marketing Assessment   147
Appendix 4: Medical Group Management Association   149
Bibliography   151

In memory of my father
Allan Bryan Cafferky, MD
1920–1953
General Practitioner

ABOUT THE AUTHOR

Michael E. Cafferky has been in the healthcare industry since 1982. He is currently the Director of Business Development for Pacific Hospital of Long Beach (California) and has worked in the past for Kettering Medical Center and National Medical Enterprises. As a consultant Mr. Cafferky has served dozens of service organizations in a variety of industries. In 1992 he traveled to Romania to serve that nation's first private, non-profit health center.

An experienced trainer, Mr. Cafferky has given speeches and seminars on word-of-mouth marketing and other marketing topics for dozens of organizations including chambers of commerce, health-care professionals, health maintenance organizations, and professional associations.

Mr. Cafferky holds advanced degrees in both public health and marketing. He is a columnist on the topic of small business marketing for *Business Tech International* magazine.

PREFACE

In 1923 an astute physician wrote a popular book entitled *The Successful Physician* (Wm. B. Saunders, Philadelphia). In that book Verlin C. Thomas, M.D., collected the best business development wisdom which had been passed down from one generation of physicians to another during the previous century. Dr. Thomas spoke in idealistic terms about how to instill confidence, faith, and gratitude in patients:

1. Listen attentively and make written notes.
2. Don't discuss finances with the patient until you have secured the patient's faith in you.
3. Display friendliness and sympathy.
4. Ask questions only about the case.
5. Make verbal observations of patient's situations before they have a chance to tell you those things themselves.
6. Explain what the diagnosis means.
7. Show patients that similar cases have responded and that you assume their cases will respond as well.
8. Live in a way that your life maintains your reputation for absolute integrity and honesty.
9. Have exemplary personal habits and clean morals.
10. Never let the fact that a patient was referred to you by another patient lead you to be careless or assume that you will keep the new patient.
11. Cultivate the most desirable personal qualities: sincerity, tact, interest, enthusiasm, intelligence, and good judgment.

Patient gratitude was the supreme emotion to which all doctors aspired. Dr. Thomas asserted that grateful patients are the greatest asset a physician can possess. Patients who are cured tend to exaggerate the seriousness of the illness and dwell on the ability of the physician. These champion patients take personal pride in the achievements of their doctors. Follow these time-tested principles, said Dr. Thomas, and you will become successful.

Dr. Thomas' book was written before the completion of the great population migration to the cities. The country doctor could move to any place that needed a physician (and most towns did), set up a modest office, and expect that people would start coming down the lane for care. Medicine was still a cash business in which physician and patient negotiated fees at the time of service.

Are our times so different that we can safely ignore Dr. Thomas' suggestions? I think not, for patients still come to the doctor's office with two conflicting feelings: anxiety about the doctor's competence and hope that the doctor will help them find a cure. For new patients, first impressions are as powerful today as they were seventy years ago. Patients still want results and action from a physician. In short, the human nature of patients, especially in regard to their personal feelings about doctors, has not changed much over the years. Ignore these and other principles and you will have a difficult time building a practice; you will risk not only your professional reputation but also your personal reputation. Follow them and you will find satisfaction and success as a medical care giver.

This book is a tactical tool that can help you make and implement a plan to build your business using just one powerful resource: your reputation in the community. Your reputation among satisfied patients is your most valuable marketing resource, something which cannot be purchased as part of a media blitz or through a high-powered marketing consultant. There is nothing in this book about strategic planning or contracting with managed care plans, nothing about hiring and firing employees, and nothing about getting on television talk shows. Instead, this book is about winning confidence, building faith, and instilling gratitude in patients who will become your loyal supporters.

If you are like every healthcare professional I have ever known, you want to build your business through the power of your reputation. Business growth through word-of-mouth marketing is a signal that you have achieved a consistent blend of art and science in your practice of medicine. This is something you hope and dream for. Using the principles in this book, it is something you can plan for and make a reality.

The book's scope is limited to one method: word-of-mouth marketing. This single-mindedness is one of its strongest features. You are not left wondering which promotional method is the best. Instead, you will find specific activities which will produce truly satisfying results.

You will find in this book the theoretical basis for word-of-mouth marketing as well as scores of practical ideas on how to make it work. Learning why word-of-mouth works will help you apply what you learn in your own setting. Another feature of the book is an emphasis on the following topics:

- How to identify the patients and people who can build your reputation

- The cost of word-of-mouth marketing

- Market segmentation

- Networking in the community

- Cross-cultural reputation building

- Training ideas to improve your internal marketing program

- How to stop negative word of mouth

- How word-of-mouth marketing fits with managed care practices

While this book can be used by large multispecialty group practices, most of its ideas can be implemented with a small staff on a low budget. No suggestions are made which require a marketing professional to help with implementation, no outside advertising agencies are needed, and no suggestions are made on how to select a marketing consultant or public relations firm. This is not to say that word-of-mouth marketing is free: it does cost time and, more important, commitment from both you and the office staff.

Other books soft-pedal the negative feelings that many physicians have toward traditional advertising. This book addresses those feelings. I hope it will persuade you not to risk violating the professional-patient relationship through inappropriate advertising. It is based on the premise that public advertising should be done only after a doctor has developed a consistent word-of-mouth marketing program and as a direct support or complement to that program.

Finally, this book offers specific ways in which the entire office can, through its own marketing effort, make a direct contribution to the overall success of the practice. The involvement of the staff in building a physician's reputation is a vital dynamic which many offices have lost sight of in the press to respond to new regulations and increased paperwork and procedures. The ideas in this book will help you get your staff members involved again.

* * *

ACKNOWLEDGMENTS

I thank my family—Marlene, Bryan, Nolan—for their support and encouragement during the research and development of my word-of-mouth marketing training programs and this book, which grew out of the seminars.

I acknowledge the many doctors and managers from Ohio to California who have, through their frank discussions with me over the last ten years, contributed practical ideas for this book. In many ways this is your book since collectively you speak with authority both to what is appropriate and to what really works in the office of a professional healthcare practitioner.

I would like to recognize the contributions of the reviewers of the Medical Group Management Association (MGMA) who, in offering their practical suggestions, have made this a better book.

Chapter 1

Reality As We Know It

The practice of medicine has changed. With the onset of new reimbursement formulas has come increased financial pressure as payments for medical services have been squeezed. Add to this price-cutting the shrinking level of health benefits available to health plan members. This frustrating process has been accompanied by a trend toward increasing demands for higher-quality care from regulators, health plans, and patients. The government has taken aggressive actions to increase the regulation of medical practices. In many cities managed care providers have taken a sizable chunk of business away from other doctors. Increases in the number of uninsured people have further eroded the patient base. Groups of doctors in metropolitan areas are getting larger, with more to spend to achieve success.

Physicians have tried many advertising tactics over the last few years, but generally with disappointing results. This experimentation has left many physicians skeptical about the value of marketing. In one of my word-of-mouth marketing training programs a physician reflected this disappointment: "I've tried the weekly shopper, door-to-door delivery, newspaper advertising, Yellow Pages, fliers, and other methods. We have managed to blow several thousand dollars and have little to show for it. I feel I've been ripped off by the advertising industry. But it won't happen again." This doctor verbalized what many feel: "You feel you must buy something, but it never works the way you expect." Doctors who have tried traditional promotional tactics are returning to the basics of word-of-mouth marketing, but many do not know how to take an organized approach to this challenge.

Many specialists have for several years maintained a small primary care practice to take care of the sore throats and upset stomachs of ultraloyal patients. They have kept this part of the practice small and invisible to the rest of the medical community. Now, however, the scene is changing. Some specialists in solo practice are quietly beginning to compete with primary care physicians for patients. A general surgeon stopped me in the physicians' parking lot and told me that to maintain his income level, he had decided to expand his practice by starting a family medicine clinic using a physician assistant. A cardiologist I heard about has decided to do the same. He now includes Pap smears in his list of services.

Does this mean doom and gloom for doctors? Hardly. There is a window of opportunity for all physicians to garner increased business by improving the quality of their services and implementing the principles of word-of-mouth marketing which successful practices have depended on for years. Now more than ever before, word-of-mouth marketing will become the central focus of the business development of a medical practice.

Doctors are realizing that their most valuable resource is their reputation with their patients in the community. While a few doctors gain national recognition among other doctors for their work, most physicians, like other professionals, are content to have a good name in the community. I have asked many doctors what gave them the most satisfaction as they were growing a business successfully. Almost without exception they all say "practicing good medicine and having my current patients recommend others to me for care." This is something which reaches into the core of what it means to be a professional: helping people and seeing that they appreciate what you do for them so much that they tell someone else.

NEGATIVE WORD-OF-MOUTH HAPPENS MORE THAN YOU THINK

One day I spoke with a patient who was coming out of a doctor's office. I asked him, "How did it go for you and did they do a good job?" His answer was revealing: "You don't go to a doctor's office and expect a good job. You just hope to survive. They see so many patients, they have little time for one in particular. Its 'What kind of insurance do you have?' 'Fill this form in, Mr. Jones,' 'What is your problem today, Mr. Jones?' 'Wait here for a minute,' 'Go in there now, Mr. Jones,' 'That will be fifty dollars, please'—with a smile. Little else is asked or said to you, but they can sure talk to each other about everything from what's for lunch to who they went out with last night after work. I don't know any more than when I came in. I guess the doctor knew what he was doing; I hope so."

Mr. Jones's case is not atypical. Up to 40 or 50 percent of patients today leave a doctor's office disappointed, disillusioned, or dissatisfied and wishing not to return to "that office." Up to 40 percent of all patients are classified as "shoppers" by doctors' offices. Some of these shoppers refuse medical advice. They seem to be on a never-ending search for the perfect doctor. Others, however, have legitimate complaints and take their patronage elsewhere. Some doctor's office employees write these patients off as simply being wacky or having unrealistic expectations. These doctor-hopping patients are seen by some doctors as pests rather than sources of opportunity to make a livelihood.

After one of my word-of-mouth marketing seminars, a medical practice manager came up to tell me about her marketing program. She said her office had been doing a word-of-mouth marketing program because almost all its patients had come by referrals from current patients. She tracks carefully where her patients come from. Her approach is to pick the best patients, encourage referrals from them, and create barriers for the undesirable patients in the hope that they will go away. "Its very easy to do," she confided. "I just tell the patients that this or that requirement is office policy, which cannot be changed for just one patient. After a while it works. They usually go away. Sometimes they get angry, but I can't help that." With this approach to weeding out undesirable patients, it is no wonder that this doctor is slowing down her practice either intentionally or unintentionally. I think she should retire now.

Unfortunately, in most metropolitan areas, most doctors do not have the luxury of having a reception room full of patients to weed through. In some cities up to 30 or even 40 percent of patients leave a doctor's office because they have a new health plan which requires them to go to someone else. Many of these patients do it without a whimper. A few do put up a fuss to their employers. They will complain about it to you and your staff. They are loyal to you. They like you. They would die for you. These, as you will see in this book, are your champion patients. Unfortunately, these patients have not been a large enough force in the market to prevent the onset of managed care, which, like it or not, is here to stay.

PERCEPTION IS REALITY

Here's a shocking statistic about dissatisfied patients. As many as 95 percent of all unhappy people will not tell a doctor that they are unhappy with the service they received. However, they are willing to tell someone else. In fact, marketing experts say that people who are unhappy with a doctor's service are ten times more likely to speak about their unhappiness to someone else than is someone who is happy with the service received. Here is another shocking point: Up to 80 percent of lost clients can be attributed to a problem with the people who work at a practice. It might be indifference, poor performance, or just a lack of the ability to get along with people. I've heard the following complaints often over the years:

1. The staff doesn't communicate clearly what is expected.
2. The nurse doesn't tell the doctor the information I give her.
3. They forget to do an important test and make me come back to the office.
4. They make me wait for hours.
5. They are more interested in office policies than in patients.
6. They don't know because they just work there.
7. They can't make any exceptions.
8. The whole office is confusing.

The list could go on until you're sick of it, but there's more. When it comes to the doctor, some patients say that physicians:

1. Prescribe medications excessively
2. Refer patients for tests too frequently

3. Don't want to spend time with them

4. Are more interested in insurance payments than in patients

5. Are selfish, arrogant, inattentive, and uninterested

Before you write off these negative perceptions as coming from a bunch of crackpot patients, consider it from their point of view. Is it in the realm of possibility that some doctors' offices create or further these negative perceptions? I can tell you for fact that these things happen. Whether you agree with these criticisms or not is irrelevant to the patient. For some patients these perceptions are reality. The question is, "What is your office doing to counteract this negative point of view?" If you are doing little or nothing, you are fighting an uphill battle against negative word-of-mouth. If you think your reputation will withstand the loss of a few negative patients, don't be so certain.

I'm not trying to engage in a subtle form of doctor bashing here. Let's not make more of this than is necessary, because these negative perceptions come from only a minority of patients. Most patients have had good or at least adequate experiences with their doctors. I encourage you to do all in your power to stop or prevent the negative perceptions and build on the positive ones. But how many patients have an exceptional experience, one that is so overwhelming that they talk about it to their friends for days?

THE POSITIVE SIDE OF WORD-OF-MOUTH

I've started with the bad news about negative word-of-mouth. It's scary to think that with so many unhappy patients roaming the streets, almost 90 percent of all new patients coming into a medical practice depended on what someone else said about the doctor. However, there is a positive side too.

As many as 70 percent of people use information from a family member or friend or from another doctor when making their selection of a doctor. Another 15 to 20 percent use information from a nurse or nonphysician health professional. A few more rely on advice from a boss. The same is true for specialists or allied health professionals to whom patients are referred by a primary care physician. Often patients rely on only a single information source when making this decision. A new patient who comes to you will probably have talked with just one person and then made up his or her mind on the basis of what that person said about you. Think about the marketing potential this has for your practice. What do you suppose that champion said about you?

Every patient who knows you also knows 200, 300, or even 400 other people. Each of those other people knows a few hundred more people. The potential total comes to hundreds of thousands of people. Closer to reality, however, there are probably three or four dozen people who know each of your patients well enough to speak with them often, and each of those other people knows three or four dozen others to talk to on a regular basis. That is great marketing leverage. Add to this the hundreds of other people who overhear a happy patient talking to a friend about his or her doctor. They stand there silently, taking it all in and evaluating their own needs for a physician. Even if they do not know the patient, they still stand there listening to that happy patient give a personal recommendation which will result in another new patient for you. Think of the marketing power you can gain by tapping into this huge grapevine.

The power of word-of-mouth extends beyond this, however, because people with characteristics similar to those of your present patients know others with similar health problems. Diabetic patients talk to one another. People with heart disease talk with each other. Mothers with small children talk to each other about the health of their children. Women having babies talk about pregnancy to women who are thinking about having babies. Men with sports injuries talk to others who have injured themselves but have not seen a doctor yet. It's human nature, and you can't stop it from happening. If you are not tapping into the power of the medical grapevine, you are spinning your promotional wheels and getting nowhere fast.

Having worked in healthcare for the last decade, I have had an opportunity to speak with many physicians about their promotional tactics. It is amazing that although most physicians believe in the power of word-of-mouth marketing, most do nothing to make sure it is happening. Very few offices have laid out word-of-mouth marketing plans for themselves. When I ask why this is true, the most common answer is, "There's not a whole lot you can do about it. If it is going to happen, it just happens." This book is written to overcome that myth. If you don't believe you can do anything about a problem, you are not likely to try. As you read this book, keep your mind open to this thought: You can do something to effect a positive word-of-mouth marketing program. You can enhance your reputation. You can see the results of happy patients talking and sending others to you.

WHAT THEY ARE TALKING ABOUT

What goes on during private conversations between champion patients and their friends or families is known only to them. Patients report, however, that when it comes to selecting a physician, the following are the most important criteria. The kind of doctor they choose

1. Seems knowledgeable

2. Seems to be interested in the patient

3. Explains what he or she is doing and why

4. Asks appropriate questions about the problem

5. Offers practical solutions for the problem

6. Spends enough time with the patient

I didn't pull these statements out of thin air. They are the issues that have been shown in the research literature to be important to patients. Other important factors in the medical research include

1. The courtesy of the office personnel

2. Whether the doctor keeps the appointment on time

3. The ability to obtain an appointment when needed

4. Responsiveness in solving problems

If all you get from this is that you and your staff should be more friendly, look more closely at the two lists above. Generating positive word-of-mouth requires much more than a smile and a warm voice. When patients come to the doctor, their primary concern is that their health problems or questions be taken care of in a competent manner so that good results occur. If the staff engages in small talk with the patient, that is not enough to convince the patient that his or her primary problem will be taken care of adequately. The other major concern is that he or she know what is happening and what will happen. In summary, patients are most interested in *competence information*.

Patients judge competence primarily by the results achieved by the prescribed treatments. They also depend on the explanations they receive, even if they do not understand everything. They notice if you are thorough in your work. If you reach a diagnosis quickly, the patient concludes that you must be competent. Patients' information needs will be satisfied if you and the staff use understandable terms in explaining procedures and medical conditions. Patients like it when you or the office nurse volunteers extra information about their health concerns. They like to have their questions answered clearly. Remember that patients without medical training may forget what they hear the first time an explanation is given. If they ask a second and a third time for an explanation, it's not because they are dumb. Medical terminology and concepts may be foreign to them. You deal with these things every day, but illness is the only time when patients really have to pay attention to medical and health issues. Being straightforward and open tells patients that you value them. Taking adequate time with a patient also contributes to the sense that you are providing the information that the patient needs.

Word-of-mouth talk is not limited to these factors. I've heard patients talk about the doctor's good-looking face, the bedside manner, the car he or she drives, the gentle voice, the level of intelligence, the hospital the doctor goes to, special areas of medical expertise, and a host of other interesting things. These other things make for great conversations with their friends. The more unusual these things are, the more interesting they are. However, good conversation pieces do not take the place of practical competence and being informative, for these two qualities are universal criteria used by all patients in all situations. Listen to what is being said about you. Let this news show you how to give better service.

PRACTICAL SUGGESTIONS IN THIS BOOK

It's nice to know that patients look for competence and information, but what can you do to encourage positive word-of-mouth? In this book I have collected a variety of practical ideas which doctors have found successful. Some of these ideas are simple to implement, requiring minimal staff training. Some are a little more involved and may require spending a small amount of money. In only a very few cases do the ideas require you to spend money. I realize that there are differences between you and some of your peers when it comes to the comfort level you feel with promotional ideas. You may feel uncomfortable with some of the activities in this book.

If this is the case, ask yourself why it is true. Is it because you are afraid of putting yourself on the line? Are your professional standards designed to enhance your reputation? Only you have to answer for your own actions, so choose those activities which fit best with your approach to practicing good medicine and your personality. If you force yourself to continue doing something that isn't right for you, you will be unhappy in your work. I encourage you to try some of the activities you at first think won't fit with your office. Leave the other activities to others who have a different approach. If you stay with what is in your opinion ethical, moral, and professional, you will be true to yourself and enjoy your career more. Here are a few ideas to start with:

1. <u>Reinforce the fact that you are competent.</u> Whenever a new patient comes in, someone in your office should make a point to tell the person that you have

   a. Successfully helped many others who have had the same condition

   b. had special training in that health problem

   c. Taken a special interest in that subject

If the staff tells the patient something like this before the patient actually talks with you, all the better. If the staff tells the patient as the patient is leaving the office, that is good too, because this is the time when the patient is developing doubts, anxiety, and curiosity about the future. A good way for the doctor to communicate competence is to tell the patient a short story about how he or she faced this same diagnosis while in residency training and has seen it many times since. Tell a few details about the patient's reaction to his or her illness and to the treatment which was prescribed. People are captivated by the human interest element, especially if it describes their own feelings about their health status before, during, and after treatment.

2. <u>Refuse to be silent.</u> Silence may be interpreted as incompetence. Give patients more information through personal conversations, written materials, conversations with their family members or guardians, telephone calls, at the reception desk—everywhere. The worst case is when you perform an examination and then disappear down the hall into another treatment room, not to be seen by the patient again that day. When this happens, patients wonder what just happened. They have anxiety about what you have found or not found. There are a lot of unanswered questions. Something close to this occurs when you simply say to the patient, "I'm giving you a prescription for this medicine. Take it twice a day for three weeks, then come back to see me" and then disappear. The next three weeks will be torture as the patient wonders what is supposed to happen, what is really wrong, and, most important, what it all means. By contrast, if you discuss the meaning of the illness, the purpose of the medication, its potential side effects, and the symptoms, you are more likely to have a happy patient who will do anything for you, including referring others.

3. <u>Let the patient know you are familiar with prior conditions which may have a direct bearing on the current situation.</u> This provides

valuable evidence that you are competent. It also confirms that you have the necessary experience to deal with the subtle differences between your patient and other patients who have the same problem. Patients are amazed when a physician can describe accurately what they are going through. They tend to believe the prognosis and accept the medical advice more quickly – and this both contributes to a positive outcome and builds your reputation.

4. Involve the patient in the discovery and treatment of the problem by asking questions, suggesting possibilities, describing similar problems, offering solutions, and discussing implications. As the patient sees the logic of differential diagnosis and your medical management, he or she will leave with a great sense of respect for your competence. This discovery process will give the patient a chance to raise other health issues. Those other health questions may be flags for other problems the patient and/or the patient's other family members are experiencing. As the patient clears the air it will enhance your diagnosis, treatment selection, and advice on follow-up care. You may even get a word-of-mouth referral out of it.

5. Reinforce the positive when your staff members evaluate a patient's experience in the office. Ask patients directly whether they felt you were competent, took enough time with them, and seemed unhurried and interested in their problems. When patients offer a statement about their level of happiness with you or the office, your staff can give them feedback based on what they think they hear the patients say. Then the staff members can clarify what they hear using their own words about which central issue the patients are most happy. Your staff may ask patients if they are pleased because of your skill and knowledge. Or was it your way with people that was most important? Going through this exercise will help your patients become champion patients sooner by defining for themselves what they like about you. When it is plain in their own minds, they will be more likely to talk about it freely to someone else.

6. Seek out the negative feelings patients exhibit in the office or hospital room. Look for subtle nonverbal cues that the patient is wondering about something, is anxious about something, is frustrated over something, or in some other way is having a negative

experience. If you see a furrowed brow, ask the patient directly what he or she is concerned about. Questions such as, "Is there something I need to know that you haven't told me?" and "You seem upset about something. Is it something I can help you with?" leave the door open for them to tell you what they are upset about.

7. <u>When someone "shops" your office on the telephone, the front staff should have a prepared script which emphasizes the most important criteria mentioned above.</u> They should tell the patient that "The doctor is knowledgeable, interested, informative," etc., as well as any specific positive things about you or the office which other patients have made a point of telling you. Your staff should never be at a loss for words to describe you in terms which patients actually use in making a selection.

Chapter 2

What it Takes to Succeed in Word-of-Mouth Marketing

I figure that if I can boil down an idea to just one or two things, I will be able to remember it. That's why I've boiled down word-of-mouth marketing to two basic issues:

1. Stopping negative word-of-mouth as much as possible, even though you can never please everyone

2. Promoting positive word-of-mouth consistently

As simple as this sounds, there is a significant amount of effort that must be put into a marketing program to help it succeed. Talking about saving money and business development won't help if your word-of-mouth marketing program is not followed carefully. Positive word-of-mouth marketing does not happen by itself. It happens because of specific skills which are consistently applied in the normal working environment with each patient.

THE THRESHOLD OF EXCELLENT SERVICE

Most patients will not say a word about you, either positive or negative, if their experience is merely adequate. If you simply meet their basic expectations they will have nothing to shout about to their friends. However, if you exceed the patient's expectations, they will find that remarkable. For each patient there is a threshold of service excellence (the place where you exceed the patient's expectations)

13

which must be crossed before positive word-of-mouth takes place. The challenge is to find this threshold during every telephone call and visit. The challenge never goes away, but it may change with changing times and changing consumer needs. As they experience excellent service, satisfied patients will gradually want more and more (it's human nature). But if they keep coming back to you and then keep talking about it to their friends, does it matter if you constantly make service adjustments? Does it matter if other people find out how well your patients are treated? Won't they get jealous and want to come to your office, too? Yes. That's the whole idea of word-of-mouth marketing: building the business with happy patients who talk about it to others. Of course, there may be limits to what you can do for patients. You have only so many hours and dollars to spend each day. Most reasonable people understand that you cannot give them the moon for a penny.

FINDING THE THRESHOLD

Your search for the threshold of excellent service can get frustrating without a few guidelines, so let me suggest two fertile areas. First, think in terms of the existing relationships between people associated with your office. Here are a few examples of relationships in which people skills offer opportunities to cross the threshold to excellent service:

Patient − doctor
Patient − nurse
Patient − manager
Patient − receptionist
Patient − billing employee
Patient − hospital staff
Patient − other patients

The list could be expanded for each different type of person in your office. The point here is that people skills is the first area that you should exceed patients' expectations. Being friendly is necessary, but it is not sufficient for the provision of excellent service. People skills require that staff members be well trained in their jobs, confident, communicative, reliable, courteous, credible, energetic, knowledgeable, attentive, and caring, with an attitude of "I can do it for you now." Positive people skills communicate to patients that you do care, are there for them and know what you are doing. If you are willing to become obsessed with positive word-of-mouth marketing, you will never be satisfied with the level of excellence in your service. You will constantly seek to improve, knowing that you can make a difference in your patients' lives.

Look at the people skills which promote positive word-of-mouth and reward them in the office. Don't be afraid to identify the people skills which make for negative word-of-mouth among patients. Begin a formal "office eavesdropping" program in which you listen to the interactions which cause frustration, anxiety, anger, disappointment, and irritation among your patients. Listen to yourself interact with people at the hospital, too. You may be surprised to find a whole new side to your personality when you talk with consultants or nurses. I've observed doctors who seem to know all the right people skills to use with patients in the office, but when they get to the hospital they turn into completely different people.

The second fruitful place to look for the threshold of service excellence is in the systems (your office procedures, policies, environment, etc.) that are in place for caring for patients from the moment they enter your business life on the telephone by making an appointment to the time when they no longer need a doctor's office. Here the key ingredients are responsiveness, efficiency, flexibility, consistency, convenience, uncomplicated procedures, reliability, accessibility, and security. For example,

1. Are your scheduling policies flexible to meet the needs of working patients?

2. Do you handle patients' finances the same way each time they visit?

3. Do you follow through on your commitments to patients?

These two areas (people skills and office systems) make up the most important qualities of the threshold of excellent service in a medical practice. Slipups in these areas can result in unhappy patients and a negative word-of-mouth. Exceeding expectations here can result in patients talking positively about you.

OTHER SUCCESS FACTORS

1. The boss. Start with yourself. Unless you are willing to employ positive word-of-mouth marketing principles, the staff will not follow. Become a proponent for word-of-mouth in your office. Become possessed by it. Practice it. Talk about it.

2. Train, train, train. We are never finished with word-of-mouth marketing. The office environment constantly changes and patient needs change too. Staff members forget the importance of people skills over time. Set a strict course of constant training and retraining until every employee improves his or her patient relations skill to the level you desire.

3. Segment the market. I'll say more about this later, but begin thinking now about how you can group your patients into meaningful categories for word-of-mouth marketing: champion patients who speak about you often and who would die for you, new patients who need an exceptionally positive experience on the first appointment (good impressions are made here), quiet patients, and patients in the larger middle group who have not shown whether they are champions.

4. Remove the barriers to positive word-of-mouth. If you have several highly specialized jobs which involve a high degree of contact with patients, do some cross-training to help your staff members do each other's work when necessary. If you are having trouble coordinating between nurses and receptionist or between nurse and doctor, eliminate this barrier. Review company policies which exist for your convenience. Change the ones you can change to help put the patient in control. Remove the indifference shown by unmotivated employees by helping them see the importance of positive word-of-mouth. Give them the power to make decisions and take actions for

patients when problems arise. Use staff meetings to conduct creative problem-solving sessions for the specific complaints which surface. Look ahead for potential problems before they become a source of irritation to patients.

5. <u>Give the champion patients more information to tell others.</u> You will read more about champion patients later in the book. For now, begin thinking about how you can keep patients informed about what is going on behind the scenes in the office. What type of information would you want to know if you had a question about the doctor?

6. <u>Give them a direct, personal experience with your office.</u> I've been a patient, and I know how impersonal a doctor's office visit can feel. In an attempt to maintain professionalism, the staff can come across as more interested in the chart than in the patient. Patients can be in your office and feel that they have not really been with you. Except for the mandatory clinical words, looks, and gestures, some feel they are ignored as persons. To prevent this type of dissatisfaction, make sure someone says something personal to the patient. Use the patient's name more than once. Ask a personal question. Look patients in the eye and speak directly to them. As obvious as this sounds, it doesn't happen in many offices.

7. <u>Give them opportunities to tell others.</u> You're not out to manipulate patients' behavior. What you want to do is help them do what they naturally enjoy doing on their own: talking about you if they believe you have a quality program. By giving them things to talk about to their friends and neighbors, you give them an opportunity to fulfill an important role in their social network. The range of possibilities here is wide. Think of it as a line graph. At one end are the direct suggestions your patients can make to others, telling them to call or make an appointment to visit you if they need a doctor. Some doctors are not comfortable with this direct approach. That is no problem, for at the other end of the graph are activities such as giving unusual or remarkable information to them which will be difficult to resist talking about to someone else. Just think how difficult it is to keep a secret. That's why marketing through the grapevine is so powerful: Almost nothing can stop it once it gets started.

8. Give them appreciation when they tell someone to make an appointment to visit your office. Genuine appreciation is always welcome, and you can't go wrong by repeating your gratitude every time a patient refers someone to you. If you need to keep confidential the fact that a certain person visited your office, you can say to your champion patient: "Our reputation is the most valuable thing we have in this community. We know you play a part in sharing this reputation with others, and we want you to know how much we appreciate that." The champion patient then says, "Oh, did Delbert Jones come to your office? I told him he should come." Your response may have to be, "In some situations we do not disclose private information about someone, and I am not free to give you details about someone who you may have referred to us; however, I do want to acknowledge your support of our reputation." The best way to do this is face to face. Place a stick-on note in the patient's chart to remind you about that patient's hard work so that the next time he or she comes in for healthcare, you can tell the patient how much you appreciate what he or she has done for you. If you know you will not see this person in your office for a long time, write a short thank you note and then thank the patient on the telephone. If you send a note or telephone a thank you, however, do not fail to thank the patient personally when you see him or her the next time. Are you worried that you won't be able to think of enough ways to show your appreciation? What if you have champion patients who send you ten, fifteen, or twenty other people who become patients? Believe me, you will find creative ways to express your thankfulness as many times as necessary.

9. Keep track of your champions. Start by making a list of the people who have referred others to you. Read that list and create a plan of action to consistently develop a personal relationship with the people on the list. This in itself will exceed the threshold of their positive expectations. If you work in a large office with a high volume of patients, remember that three or four of every ten patients may be champion-type patients. Getting to know who they are is step one. Maintaining a positive personal relationship is step two. If you need to divide up the champion list because of the high volume, get several

people in the office involved in keeping track of champions. Think of it this way: If all other forms of promotion were withdrawn from you except word-of-mouth marketing, how closely would you maintain contact with your champions? These relationships with the people who speak for you in the community would become the most important to you, and you would do just about anything ethical and legal to maintain your good reputation and their good favor.

10. <u>Start small and stay focused.</u> When you initiate a word-of-mouth marketing program, begin with the basic elements and then embellish the program. Follow this outline as a guide:

a. <u>Identification</u>: Identify by name the patients who are responsible for your reputation; make and keep current a written list.

b. <u>Encouragement</u>: Pick one or two ideas you can implement on a consistent basis that will promote your reputation and get patients to continue talking for you.

c. <u>Gratitude</u>: Pick one or two methods of showing gratitude when your loyal supporters refer others to the practice.

Chapter 3

Word-of-Mouth Marketing Theory

Don't be fooled by the title of this chapter. There are several great word-of-mouth marketing ideas here which can be implemented in a healthcare practice. If you are bored by theory, skip this part. However, if you are curious about how word-of-mouth marketing works and why it works the way it does, read on. When you do, you will probably think of things you can do to promote positive word-of-mouth. Even if you skip this part, you may want to look at the last few of pages of this chapter to get a summary of practical ideas. After all is said and done by the marketing experts, it is what works that counts.

There are some things about word-of-mouth marketing which scientists simply don't know. It just works. Most marketing experts I know believe that word-of-mouth is by far the most effective way to communicate with consumers. Other than direct contact, word-of-mouth from a happy patient is the most personal and therefore, the most powerful form of communication.

If you want to hang on your wall a reminder of the most basic principles of word-of-mouth marketing, put up two simple words that summarize everything: *PEOPLE TALK.*

We all talk, but social scientists know that some people talk and are listened to more than others. Who are the talkers who get listened to in your practice? Essentially, they are the ones who are perceived to be believable, genuine, experienced, and interested in what they are talking about. If someone can document that he or she has had a recent experience with your practice (this can be done by saying, "Last week I went to my doctor."), he or she is more likely be listened to and believed. If one of your patients talks with enthusiasm, he or she will more likely be heard. Enthusiasm is a sign of being genuine.

Also, if a patient appears not to have an axe to grind on behalf of your practice, it adds to that patient's believability. All these factors build the talker's credibility. Other factors which add to credibility include being familiar with the information one talks about, using persuasive arguments to convince others of the truth of what one says, and whether those who listen have had good results from following a person's advice in the past.

People who spread your good reputation to others are self-confident and innovative, willing to try new products and services. They can be observed talking a lot about similar products, services, or related products (anything in healthcare or personal care will do just fine for them). They have many friends and talk a lot about people they know; in other words, they have a high degree of social interaction all the time. Finally, they talk primarily with people in a similar age group or socioeconomic setting.

What does this mean for your practice? It simply means that you need to begin identifying people who spread your reputation. Start by finding the patients who

1. Have already referred others to you (this is the most important indicator)

2. Are naturally outgoing and sociable

3. Have recent experience with your office

4. Have a lot of detailed information about your practice and the people who work there

5. Have a natural enthusiasm when speaking

6. Speak convincingly

7. Are in positions of leadership in a family, company, club, or community (they didn't get in to these positions without having people listen to them)

8. Are socially mobile, that is, have a car or ride public transportation often

9. Read magazines or other materials dealing with products of interest

10. Exhibit a high degree of interest in a product or service in the same category

11. Show personal interest in your practice through questions and comments

12. Have demonstrated personal gratitude for your excellent service, calling on the telephone to tell you, writing a thank you note, or saying something directly to you in the office

13. Report to you that others turn to them for help in difficult situations

You may not be able to apply all these factors equally to all patients, but use your best judgement and identify by name those who are the most likely candidates. Have your staff help by making a list of people to whom others listen. Don't think about longterm patients only; your best promoters can be new patients. What you are looking for among your patients is leadership: those to whom others listen.

HOW LEADERS CREATE SUCCESS FOR YOU

Marketing experts call this process of people talking and getting listened to *opinion leadership*. Such leadership is the backbone of successful word-of-mouth marketing efforts. Scientists have found that opinion leaders are not necessarily perceived as leaders in everything but are considered opinion leaders for specific products or services. In other words, your patients may not be seen as experts in buying motor homes or television sets, but because of their experience in health care, they know doctors and hospitals pretty well. They can talk convincingly about the differences between doctors' offices because they have personal experience.

Opinion leaders help a business succeed by giving helpful information to their listeners. You may be surprised at the specific details these leaders remember from their experience in your office which can be helpful to prospective patients: how to get an appointment when they really need one, how well the doctor responds to their health problems, etc. They also remember a host of other things which can be supportive or damaging to word-of-mouth including the color of the drapes and carpet, the comfort of the chairs in the reception room, the temperature of the vinyl exam table, the smells in the back office, and whether the office is cluttered.

Opinion leaders help prospective patients by reducing the time they need to spend searching for information about a new doctor. With their own personal experience as evidence, they reduce the perceived risk of trying a new doctor. A prospective patient may know you exist by knowing your name and seeing you listed in the telephone book, but an opinion leader will help shape the attitudes of prospective patients just before they make the decision whether to call your office.

Reports from opinion leader patients help new patients by giving them inside information that is not accessible anywhere else. These details are often the most valuable in decision making because they focus on your personal side. If your loyal supporters repeat information new patients have heard in other places, it confirms for the new patients the value of getting care from your office. If what the new patient hears is different from what he or she hears in other places, the words of your supporter will help the new patient compare carefully before making a decision.

Patients who talk for you give a lot of information to others both actively and passively. If they have an exceptional experience at your office or with a service you provide, they are likely to actively talk about you to others who don't even ask. They also talk about you when asked questions such as, "what is your doctor like?" "Do you have a good doctor?" and "Do you know a good doctor I could go to?"

NEW PATIENTS USE OPINION LEADERS TO MAKE DECISIONS

Deciding on a new doctor involves a complex set of thoughts and actions. When a person first becomes aware of you or your practice, that person may use printed promotional materials or advertising to learn about your practice. During this phase of decision making patients rely on their own resourcefulness to find information. When they begin evaluating the information about you, most people rely on word-of-mouth for most of the details; advertising or paid promotion plays a much smaller role.

The next step in the decision model occurs when the patient is ready to decide whether to call your office. Looking for a new physician involves a high degree of mental energy and interest. It is not a decision to take lightly. That's why during this phase a new patient looks to others to help him or her evaluate the possibilities.

Immediately after making a decision, new patients begin to rely on their own experience. The report of a happy patient means little to them except in the sense that the report they received set them up to think positively about their encounter with you. Now they rely almost exclusively on their own judgment of their personal experiences. The first few minutes in the office and then with you are the most crucial to them in developing lasting impressions. Then, as time passes, they gradually put more stock in what advertising and printed information say and the words of happy patients to inform their judgment. Their own experience eventually takes over as the primary contributor to your reputation.

You may guess from this that the most important time to have opinion leaders talk with prospective patients is when these people are evaluating their options. They most likely have a felt need for a physician and have begun the search. If a loyal patient speaks with them about you, there is a high probability that the new patients will seek your care.

Immediately after making the decision to come to you for care, new patients rely almost exclusively on their own experience to judge your reputation as presented by a champion patient. Thus, it is clear that first impressions build a doctor's reputation. If new patients are treated with respect and go away with a sense that you cared, their anxiety will dissipate quickly and they will feel good about the decision. Therefore, it is important that new patients be overwhelmed with good service, something which some medical practices do not try to accomplish. Also, there appears to be room for advertising (promotion) of some type to help in the confirmation process. Written information about you, such as a resume, copies of thank you letters from happy patients, and other forms of promotion, can help new patients feel satisfied that they made the right decision in coming to you.

WHY WOULD AN OPINION LEADER TALK ABOUT YOU?

Opinion leader patients don't get money for bringing in new patients. If you follow through carefully with them, they will receive a sincere thank you for their work. So why do they bother to talk about the practice? What's in it for them? First, opinion leaders get an enormous amount of personal satisfaction from being listened to and looked up to. They enjoy being a point of reference for others. It helps them gain attention, enhances their status, and helps them assert their superiority and demonstrate their awareness and expertise. But what do you care if they get psychological goodies from talking to others about your practice? It doesn't matter as long as these opinion leaders have had a good experience with your practice and have successfully referred other patients who also have a positive experience.

Second, these practice champions usually get highly involved with your practice (remember that they like to get inside information about the practice and take their experience with you seriously). High involvement means they must tell someone about it. When asked, they can't help themselves: they have to talk. Talking about your practice is a way they can enjoy social interaction with others. In other words, talking about you becomes pleasurable in itself because of the social interaction.

WHY DO FOLLOWERS LISTEN?

Between 20 and 40 percent of the population can be considered opinion leaders. This means that the rest of the population either follows the advice of others or is staunchly independent and follows its own course. Why do the rest follow? Making a decision on whether to go to a doctor means serious involvement for some people. They have a difficult time predicting what you will behave like, how they will take to the office system, and how the finances will be handled. Deciding on you as their doctor can be a relatively complex issue for many people. As the complexity increases, so does the likelihood that they will seek outside information from someone who knows you—someone with personal experience. The greater the involvement in the decision, the greater the chance that they will talk to someone, ask that person's opinion, and follow the advice they receive.

It is difficult to "test drive" an experience with your office. Furthermore, patients cannot easily use objective facts with which to make their own judgments of you until after they have had an experience in the office. They need the trusted personal influence of a friend or associate to help them do what they cannot do for themselves. There's nothing wrong with being socially dependent on others for information and advice. It's part of our culture. We all are dependent some of the time for some products.

WHEN DOES YOUR REPUTATION SPREAD?

Practice champions are just like everyone else: They talk in normal social situations. You know how conversations go. Someone begins with one topic, and after a few minutes someone mentions another topic related to the first. I call this phenomenon *conversation swing*. Usually people talk about people: what happens to people or something involving people. (What else is there to talk about?) When the topic of conversation naturally swings toward your practice, an opinion leader patient will think of it. It's human nature. Sure, you cannot control when they think and talk positively about your practice because you don't know when or where it happens. But it does happen because these people talk all the time to friends and associates. They talk to other people in church, in a club, at work, in the neighborhood, and in a recreation group. Most often, they talk to their families. When their house doors are shut and these opinion leaders are alone with their family, they may be the most honest about what they experienced in your practice. And their family members talk to their friends, associates, club members, and other family members.

Positive messages about you also spread as prospective patients observe the nonverbal communications of your champion patients. This is most often the case with immediate family members who have close contact with a champion patient before, during and immediately after a visit to your office. Their reactions to how they were treated and their emotional states are indicators of their judgment of your service. Sometimes a family member doesn't have to say anything but is upset about something that happened in your office. Their emotions rise to the surface as soon as they get near people they can let their hair down with.

SUMMARY

Word-of-mouth marketing is an informal communication process in which the champion patient does not speak professionally on your behalf. These opinion leaders are highly persuasive because they are perceived as having nothing to gain from their positive words. Word-of-mouth marketing is usually a face-to-face communication event, the most powerful form of communication. If you want a practice which is based 90 percent on referrals, you will do what successful professionals have been doing for years: follow these marketing tactics. Unlike traditional direct mail marketing, where you simply arrange for someone to send a message uninvited to someone's home, word-of-mouth marketing is highly personal, although it demands a continual obsession to make it work. Word-of-mouth marketing is never done. You cannot simply assign it to an outside marketing consultant. It is a constant, unrelenting opportunity to build a practice.

One doctor I spoke with said that he believed that the ideas I had been gathering over the years should be applied to all patients, not just opinion leaders. "We should be giving all our patients the same level of attention that you suggest we give to opinion leaders," he said. To his surprise, I agreed.

PRACTICAL IDEAS TO IMPLEMENT THE THEORY

1. <u>List your champions for all the staff to see</u>. Have a staff meeting to read the list and discuss it internally. These champions should be on everyone's mind to stress how important they are for word-of-mouth marketing. Have the list available for quick reference and easy editing when a new talker surfaces. If your scheduling system is computerized make a note or put a flag next to each patient who is identified as a talker so that you know when those patients are due to come into the office. When you schedule an opinion leader for an office visit or hospital visit, inform the staff about the appointment schedule and then overwhelm the patient with excellent service when he or she comes in.

2. <u>Identify other opinion leaders who are not your patients but who know you or know about you and can talk to others</u>. If you take word-of-mouth marketing seriously, you will want to know these people by name. You will know the professionals in the same building or down the block, the pharmacist, the shoe repairer, the clerk in the dress shop, and anyone else who is an opinion leader in the community. Make a list of these people and begin planning specific activities to generate enthusiasm in their talk about you. Drop in to say hello when you go out for lunch; better yet, invite them to lunch sometimes. Let them have a few coupons for the free or discounted services you give only to opinion leader patients. These people can pass the positive word along just as well as patients can. Invite them in for a tour of the office and introduce them to the staff. Celebrate when they come in and then send a personal thank you note in appreciation for their time and support.

3. <u>Give more information to your opinion leaders about the practice and its personnel</u>. If you need to, make a master checklist of the

types of information you want all your champions to know. Each time an opinion leader comes in for visit, make sure to share more information with that person. This not only is interesting to them, it gives them something else to talk about when they leave the office. If you were mentioned in the news recently, give them a copy of the news clipping. If you have published a professional paper, mention it. If the office nurse received an award from his or her peers, mention it. If someone gets married, mention it. Make sure every patient has a chance to read your resume at least once. Post it in the reception room in a nice picture frame.

4. Identify the reputation builders. Ask your patients what similar products or services they are interested in and give them more information about these too. If they are interested in home water treatments for their feet, they are likely to talk about this (and about you) with their friends. If they watch health programs on the local cable television station, make sure to stock current copies of a program guide listing their favorite shows. Create a short checklist of health, safety, beauty, and personal care issues and have a stock of magazine article reprints to hand out or some verbal information to give on those issues. Pharmaceutical suppliers and product manufacturers can supply a lot of written materials to support this effort. Pharmaceutical sales reps and hospital librarians can even do some of the legwork in researching magazine articles to present to patients. Even if the topics are not interesting to you personally, you are helping these opinion leaders do their work better as they use you as a credible information source to quote or refer to. Your office will be looked to as the place to go for expert information. More important, this provides another natural conversation swing opportunity.

5. Look for innovators among your patients. Remember that these patients are most likely the opinion leaders. Ask your patients when they last tried a new over-the-counter medicine or new health and beauty aid product. Ask them which one. Ask them if they often try new products. You are looking for an opportunity to have them talk to their friends about a new product and about you. Ask a supply house to give you some marketing samples of a product you can use

in word-of-mouth marketing and give the product to your patients as a sample to test.

6. <u>Never forget word-of-mouth marketing leaders</u>. When a practice champion passes away, be sure to attend the funeral. These patients leave behind a legacy of people who know you through their patients' experience. Don't avoid this opportunity to extend positive word-of-mouth by missing the funeral. This patient was a valuable resource for you and they should be honored.

7. <u>Always go with patients who have responded before</u>. The most likely candidates for champion patients are those who have already referred others to you. A psychology professor once told me that the best predictor of future behavior is past behavior. If you have to rank your champion patient list, put at the top those who have already referred patients. If you have limited resources to spend on word-of-mouth marketing, start by spending those funds on patients who have championed your practice in the past. It is the champion patients who build your reputation.

8. <u>When you make changes based on suggestions, always tell your champion patients how you have improved the system</u>. This is another variation on keeping patients informed and it shows that you take suggestions and complaints seriously. Simply placing a small typewritten notice at the reception desk, in the exam room, or by the suggestion box will keep patients informed about how you have responded to their suggestions.

9. <u>It's okay to ask patients who they rely on or how often others rely on them for advice regarding medical products and services</u>. Do others regard them as a good source of information on health care? How often do other people ask them for their opinion? The answers to these questions will help you identify the leaders.

10. <u>The socially isolated are the least likely to be opinion leaders</u>. However, a moral issue is involved in providing the same quality of care for the isolated and the other nonopinion leaders as well as for the mobile. If you make a point of serving those with the least access to care, you can leverage this community service to your advantage if your champion patients know about it. Let them know what type of

community service you do to help the socially isolated the next time these champions come into the office. Post a notice, mention it verbally, or put a thank you note in your hall of fame set.

11. <u>Spend time finding more situations in which the conversation swing can move to your advantage</u>. Here are a couple of ideas:

    a. Discuss a magazine article or videotape with a champion patient and then give a copy to the patient to give to someone else.

    b. Send direct mail to champions, informing them about new things in your practice: new systems, new procedures, and new treatment protocols which benefit themselves and their friends. Ask them to ask someone else's opinion about the matter and report back to you on it.

12. <u>Pick out the cream of the crop from your list and take them to dinner</u>. Specialists who depend on referrals from primary care doctors have been doing this for years. You can host such a dinner in a restaurant or even at your home, whichever is more comfortable. Allow plenty of time for informal talk at the dinner, making sure to talk with each person personally before, during, or after the meal. Then make a formal presentation (you can even read a prepared script) recognizing each guest separately for what he or she has added to the practice. If you talk without a script, have someone from the office take notes on the specific things you say about each patient. If you need help generating this presentation, ask the staff members for their ideas. This formal presentation is a natural time to tell all the patients that you value their support and that what they say about your practice is important. Follow the meal with a personal thank you note summarizing what you appreciate about each patient. These notes can be drawn from the script you read or, better yet, from the actual scripts themselves; this is a powerful way to say thank you and is a lot less expensive than buying gifts. I sat in a dinner where this type of appreciation was shown to a small group, and I could feel the appreciation that was generated.

13. <u>Give new product samples to a select group of opinion leaders/ champions and ask them to talk about the product to their friends</u>

and family members. Ask them to report back to you about the responses they get. These could be new products which you can get from the manufacturer at no charge if you tell the manufacturer the type of word-of-mouth marketing experiment you are conducting. Or they could be existing products (again donated by a manufacturer or supplier) that are available on the retail level. As a last resort, you can even describe new product ideas you or your staff read about in journals or heard about from associates. Ask the patients for a commitment to talk about the product and report back to you. When they report back, ask with whom they spoke. This will give you an indication of the types of people these champions talk with. If they come to the office for a visit and have not reported back on the product, remind them about their commitment and let them know you are interested in what they find. Why will this help you? You couldn't care less about the reactions to the product they talk about. What you are doing is creating a natural conversation swing toward a topic you want them to talk about with their friends: you and your practice.

14. Play the practice trivia game. One month a year or one week a month conduct a trivia quiz to determine which patients know the most about your practice. This paper and pencil quiz can be implemented in the reception room. It serves two purposes: It will tell you who has the most knowledge about the practice (remember that those who know more about your practice have more to say and will be listened to more often), and it will give more information to patients who don't know very much about the practice but would be eager to talk about you if they knew more. Pick interesting tidbits of personal information which add credibility to your practice. Include things such as

   a. The educational background of key medical personnel
   b. Special awards or recognition received
   c. How long the practice has been serving the community
   d. How many families with at least two generations are in the practice
   e. Community service
   f. Difficult cases you have been successful in treating
   g. A few humorous bits of trivia as long as they are in good taste and cannot be used as negative word-of-mouth

People like trivia games and like to have this information when they talk to their friends. Reward patients who get high scores on the trivia games by

a. Personally commenting on how well they did
b. Asking them how they learned so much about the practice (you will find out more helpful word-of-mouth marketing information here)
c. Giving them a complimentary gift
d. Sending them a personal note acknowledging their high scores and reinforcing the value of this knowledge for the practice

Making up trivia games can be fun for the entire staff. (This will help inform the staff members too and add credibility in their eyes.) It does take time, but the payoff of well-informed patients will be enormous. Make sure you get to see each version of your practice trivia game before the patients do.

15. Conduct more thorough research on your patients' social networks when it feels appropriate. Having strong social support groups is a way people adjust to stress (including illness). A strong social network is also an indication that a patient is an opinion leader or knows a few opinion leaders. To help you determine the strength of a patient's social network, inquire about the patient's family and close friends. Ask questions such as

a. Do you have regular, consistent contact with other people in your community? What types of groups or people?
b. Among the people you know, including yourself, who are some of the most capable, active individuals who are concerned with healthcare?
c. Who would you pick to represent your circle of friends in a discussion about healthcare (you may include yourself)?
d. Do you invite people over for parties or just to relax at your house?
e. Are you involved with any clubs or organizations? Do you hold an office or lead in some way? What type of work do you do for that group?

f. How much do you find other people coming to you for advice on health matters? Do you find that you have a lot to say about personal health?

g. Do you sometimes wish you had more information about your health?

Take note of the types of family members and friends they are most likely to talk to. Take into account the patient's age, social setting, proximity of residence, offspring, siblings, gender, etc. If you find some patients who are in large, extended families and are the family matriarch or patriarch, consider honoring them with a family dinner where the whole family attends and make the event similar to item 12 on page 31. If your patient is not the matriarch or patriarch, ask the patient to bring this important person in so you can meet him or her personally. When this opinion leader comes in, celebrate by giving him or her the grand tour and introductions to the staff. Tell this matriarch or patriarch how much you appreciate having his or her offspring as a patient.

16. Find ways to thank patients who support your positive reputation. You can hardly go wrong with verbal and written statements of gratitude. When it comes to gift giving, however, be careful not to give a present that is too expensive. If the value of your gift is, in the mind of your patient, too high for what the patient has done for you, the patient may think you are just trying to get something else instead of genuinely expressing gratitude. If you choose to use a gift giving program to thank those who support your reputation, make the gifts modest. I'll say more about showing gratitude later.

* * *

Two simple principles constitute the theory behind word-of-mouth marketing: People talk. Packed into these two principles, however, are your most valuable professional possessions as a care giver. Care for these assets with the same dedication you feel toward your patients and you will succeed in marketing.

Chapter 4

Patient Power with Clusters of People

As a doctor, you will find it almost impossible to engage in mass marketing. Only a large medical group serving a wide geographic area should consider mass marketing. Instead of trying to be all things to all people, select small groups of patients you can serve well. This process of selecting small, definable groups and then concentrating marketing resources on them is called *market segmentation*.

To be more efficient and effective, healthcare marketers have been trying for years to put patients into groups that have similar needs or characteristics. For example, children have needs different from those of geriatric patients, and diabetic patients have needs different from those of cardiac patients. We have tried grouping patients by age, gender, diagnosis, geographic location and several other categories. These are valid ways to segment or cluster the market into meaningful groups which represent business opportunities. This approach helps us save money and helps us get better at meeting the needs of specific patients.

It doesn't matter which of these methods you use as long as your choice makes business sense. There have to be enough people in the group to make a difference. They have to have purchasing power (decision-making authority, money, and experience in making decisions). Finally, you have to be able to find them to communicate with them.

These approaches, however, miss the point of word-of-mouth marketing because opinion leaders can be found in all segments of society and in every cluster that can be created for marketing purposes. The fact that people have diabetes, live in a certain ZIP code, or are over age sixty-five may have little to do with whether they talk about your practice to others: some do, and some do not. To be effective in word-of-mouth marketing, then, you need to think differently about market segmentation. You need a whole new set of categories based on the word-of-mouth needs patients have in regard to opinion leadership.

This doesn't mean that you should throw out all your ideas for dealing with the traditional groups of patients you serve. The needs presented by each of these groups do not go away just because you are organizing a consistent word-of-mouth marketing program. This means that for word-of-mouth marketing on a day-to-day basis, you must think differently about everyone connected with the practice. I recommend that you restructure your entire marketing approach by beginning with the word-of-mouth marketing segments and building from there to include the other, more traditional clusters.

WHAT ARE THE PRIMARY WORD-OF-MOUTH CLUSTERS?

There are several logical word-of-mouth marketing groups, including the following:

1. Quiet patients

2. New patients

3. Established/loyal patients

4. Opinion leader/champion patients

5. Opinion leader/champion nonpatients

Each group requires the same basic marketing tactics: (1) providing excellent service to build positive word-of-mouth, (2) quick and responsive complaint-handling procedures to stop negative word-of-mouth, and (3) more information to give to others. I am not suggesting that a different quality of care be given to patients who you know are telling others about you. As a professional, you should give every patient the same high standard of care without regard to the patient's social or cultural characteristics. Remember that patients who seem to be silent types can be opinion leaders in their own environment. What is different for each group of patients is the emphasis you place on them for word-of-mouth and what you can do to get them motivated to talk about your practice when the time is right.

QUIET PATIENTS. As was noted above, the most important patients are those who are opinion leaders, who extend your reputation. But not all patients appear to be reputation builders; indeed, many come to be patients simply because they listen to others. They have had good success following the advice of opinion leader patients, and now they have come to your practice. Don't assume, however, that there is nothing to do with this group in regard to word-of-mouth marketing. If one of these patients comes to your practice and has a horrible experience, he or she can easily begin producing volumes of negative word-of-mouth. These patients can be silent but deadly if you cross them. Also, just because they seem to be the quiet type in the reception room, this doesn't mean they are introverted. You may not know it yet, but they could be sleeping champions who are not showing it yet. They may appear to be introverts in the office, but outside they blossom into word-of-mouth champions. What should you do with quiet patients? You can do the following:

1. Keep them coming back by providing excellent service.

2. Resolve complaints quickly to prevent negative word-of-mouth.

3. Look for more evidence that they are opinion leaders in a field other than healthcare. If they are opinion leaders in purchasing another service, you may still have an opportunity to include them as opinion leaders.

4. Refuse to take them for granted.

NEW PATIENTS. New patients probably relied on the word of other people when deciding to come to your office. Now, however, they put these personal recommendations aside and begin judging for themselves. You feel good about having a new patient come: You feel you have succeeded in your marketing efforts. You are looking forward to having a good proportion of these new patients turn out to be champions. However, they look at things differently. During the first few visits they are in a "wait and see" mode.

Even if they received a glowing report from a champion patient, their anxieties shoot up when they come to the office. The more difficult they perceive their own health problems to be, the more anxiety they feel. If the forms they have to fill out are confusing, they feel anxious. If being in a physician's office is a new experience, this adds to their anxiety. The anxiety also increases if it seems to take longer than expected to get well.

Remember that new patients often have multiple health concerns. If they do not present all these concerns during the first visit, it is because they are checking you out to see how you do. Some patients intentionally give only a partial description of their symptoms to see how thorough the doctor is or how accurate he or she is in making a diagnosis. These patients represent a source of repeat business if you are careful in your work.

Here are some suggestions that apply equally well to first-time walk-in patients and to new patients with appointments:

1. <u>Have your staff acknowledge new patients enthusiastically upon their arrival</u>. A smile is not enough. A patient should be greeted with enthusiasm by the receptionist. Instruct your staff to do the following things. Personally assist the patient in completing the patient questionnaire in a private room. Serve the patient coffee, tea, or another drink. Use the patient's name frequently in conversation. Take at least sixty seconds and get to know the patient and learn who his or her significant others are (family members and friends are all potential patients). Take another sixty seconds and give a scripted description of how the office works, the complaint seeking and handling system, and the commitment to quality service. Be sure to thank patients for entrusting their care to your office. Ask who they spoke with before deciding to come to the doctor. It is not enough to ask, "How did you hear about the practice?" You want to find out the names of current patients who refer their friends to your office. If a patient does not mention significant other people, ask a couple of questions based on what you see in the patient

questionnaire to find out who they are likely to talk to as a result of the visit to the doctor. People talk. Key in on one or two feelings they have and do your best to verbalize how you would feel if you were in that situation, but do not simply say, "I understand how you feel." This is a sure sign that you are not sure how they feel or do not know how to verbalize your understanding. Finally, explain that the physician must have a few minutes to look through the patient questionnaire so that he or she will be better prepared to perform the medical service. This helps the patient understand the reason for a slight delay in seeing the physician. Explain that whenever they have a question about what is said to them or about anything else, they can ask the doctor at any time.

2. Give plenty of reassurance if you see signs of anxiety. Talk to the patient. Ask patients how they feel about being in the office. Let them know that you and the staff are there to help with any part of the experience, including paperwork, questions they may have after they go home, and how things work in the office.

3. Begin looking for referrals. This should be done discreetly, not aggressively. The intake form should have a space for the patient to make a referral. It simply asks: "Does anyone you know have a health problem that he or she is not taking care of right now and whom you would like to see get relief?" You can personalize this question to the type of specialty your office emphasizes. If the patient answers yes on the form, make note of this in the exit interview and give the patient a chance to tell you who he or she is thinking of, or give the patient a practice brochure to take to the person he or she is considering for a referral to the practice. Why would you ask a new patient for a referral? Simply because people with health problems often speak with other people who have similar problems. People talk. By the end of the first visit, the patient will be overwhelmed by how well he or she is being treated and will probably be thinking of someone else who would enjoy the same treatment. Why not give the patient a chance to respond immediately? Never pressure a patient for this information. Patients will give it if they are ready. If they do not, no problem. They will have another chance to give the information later, when they are more comfortable.

4. Give the grand tour of the office introducing the new patient to all the staff members. Introduce the patient by name each time (pronounce the name correctly early to show you care). Celebrate the new patient. If you can find out early who referred the patient to you, emphasize this to all the staff members when you introduce the patient saying: "I'd like you to meet Martha Jones, a new patient who was referred by Jane Norris." This way you are emphasizing several things at once: the new patient, the referring patient, and the role the staff plays in creating happy patients who send others to you.

5. As soon as the patient is finished with the questionnaire, have a staff member show the patient to the exam room and give him or her a personal copy of your resume just before you come in. Having positive information about you before the first exam will increase the chances that a patient will have a positive experience. It helps reduce anxiety. It builds positive expectations and trust in your competence.

NOTE: Your resume should provide knowledge a new patient lacks. If they have more knowledge about you, patients will want to refer more friends and family members. You may have a copy of your resume posted in the reception area. However, new patients may not have had to spend more than a few seconds in the reception area before they were whisked to a private room to complete the patient questionnaire. Ideally, the resume the patient receives should be on one small page (the size which can fit in a purse, a pocket, or a standard business envelope). You may want to have your photo or a photo of the entire staff on the resume (some new patients will not have seen you before and will feel more comfortable if they have a chance to see what you look like before the visit). The resume should emphasize the accomplishments which show you are credible and competent. Educational background, awards, professional affiliations, patriotic service, and community service are all sources of information to put on the resume. Do not list specific academic publications with heavy scientific language in the titles unless they are important for the specific treatments you provide on a regular basis. You can also include a short statement that the doctor is accepting new patients and that you welcome referrals.

6. <u>Fix one exam room for new patients and give them a few minutes to enjoy it before they meet you</u>. Loyal patients can be sent to this room once in a while to refresh their memory. Here's how you can do it:

a. Post thank you notes from happy patients on the wall of the exam room. These are testimonials to the competence of and the care received in the office.

b. Place your resume on a larger-than-life poster on the wall. This professionally done poster should include a color portrait of yourself, a smaller group portrait of the entire staff, and snap shots of the staff in action with patients.

c. On a bulletin board, post before and after photos of successful cases you have treated if these cases involved a cosmetic or major visual improvement in the patients.

d. Put up another professionally done poster or sign showing your personal commitment to patients and stating the guarantee you offer, the promises you make, your policy on solving problems and making things right, and an acknowledgment that most of your patients come because of the reputation that other patients have created for you in the past.

e. If you have given speeches or published articles or books, place cover sheets, title pages, or other representations of these accomplishments in picture frames. Hang them on the wall in an attractive grouping.

f. Have a separate corner or section of the wall to show photos of your involvement in the community: your participation in the Little League team, your work on the local charity, and your service to the Cancer Society and all other major high-visibility organizations. Make sure to place captions under the framed photos that describe who, what, where, and why.

g. Have one section in the room, maybe a tabletop display, where you list all your services in terms patients can understand. If you provide free services, list them prominently with a note signed by you that encourages all new patients to ask for those services.

7. <u>If there is a suggestion box in the exam room, explain what it is for</u> <u>and tell the patients that they will have a few minutes after the exam/</u> <u>treatment to complete one of the cards.</u> Emphasize how getting information like this helps you maintain a high-quality service for them and their family members and friends.

8. <u>After the exam, take an extra minute to tell your patients how</u> <u>much you appreciate the opportunity to serve them and that no</u> <u>matter what their health problems are, you are glad they came to</u> <u>you.</u> Be sure to refer to the patient by name at least twice.

9. <u>Conduct all financial conversations in a private setting rather than in</u> <u>the hallway, where staff members and other patients can hear.</u> This sets up a positive trust that you will listen to them carefully. If they ever have a complaint, you can discuss the matter in the private consultation room.

10. <u>Make sure the final good-bye is given formally by the manager or</u> <u>nurse.</u> If you have a "new patient gift" program, this is the time to present the gift. Ask patients if they have any questions about the next steps to follow for their health or about the office procedures. *Note*: Does all this take time? Yes. No one ever said excellent service in the medical field is quick and easy. It is hard work, and you can never lower your level of professionalism. Your first job with new patients is to get them to want to return to the office as often as necessary. Your second job is to so overwhelm them with excellent service that they cannot help but tell someone else about the practice. If new patients are seen as potential referral sources, the little extra time spent with them is well worth it. Remember that word-of-mouth marketing isn't free. It does cost the practice something, but it is the most natural, cost-effective, and productive way to build the business and enhance the professional-patient relationship.

11. <u>Record on charts or tracking forms the marketing information</u> <u>about who patients talked with when deciding to come to your of-</u> <u>fice.</u> Make notes in patients files on who you think the significant people are in their life and who they are likely to talk with after the visit. Also, make note of the specific company where a patient or patient's spouse works. Here is another natural network of friends

and associates to whom someone (the patient or the family member) will probably talk. These people are as significant as the patient in the word-of-mouth process which follows. If you find a new company from which you have never received any patients before, make a special effort to turn that particular patient into a champion who will work for you.

12. Send follow-up letters to whoever referred the patient to your practice and to the patient. The thank you for your referral letter should be as carefully crafted as any marketing letter. Even if it is hand-written on a note card, it should be well thought out in advance. Sample thank you letters can be kept on file to speed up the writing. The welcome to the practice letter is important too. Make it personalized to each patient's situation even if you draw upon some form letters you have used in the past.

13. Do something completely astounding. Call a new patient on the telephone the next evening. The call must be kept short, with a tidbit of information, a lab result, a reminder about a key part of your medical advice, or simply a statement that you are interested in the patient's health and are glad the patient chose to come to the office.

14. Don't reprimand new patients for taking so long to call the office, not giving you a complete medical history or the current symptoms, or not following the advice of other physicians. If their health status has deteriorated because of delay or noncompliance, you can inform patients about this without punishing them in the process.

15. Ideas for new patient gifts:

Copy of a health or leisure magazine

Coffee mug

Magnetic refrigerator note pad

Health video (on loan)

Coupon for free or discounted exam for a friend

Sample pharmaceuticals or other medical products

16. Give patients helpful information on how to use the office and on other resources. These resources include the hospital, the medical

equipment company, the pharmacist, or home nursing care. Write up half-page explanations of the following:

   a. What to do when someone you know needs a doctor
   b. When you should call the doctor's office
   c. When you should use the emergency room at the hospital
   d. What to ask the pharmacist
   e. How home nursing can help
   f. What you should know about going to the hospital for inpatient services
   g. What you should know about going to the hospital for outpatient services
   h. How to find out what your health plan covers
   i. How to get information about Medicare or Medicaid

You will think of other ideas, too. If you want to dress them up on high-quality paper with a simple but tasteful graphic design, so much the better. The next best choice is to generate these notes using a word processor and a laser printer. If you use clean paper with letter-quality print, you are performing the same valuable service. Avoid making photocopies of photocopies, however, since this usually adds unsightly black specks to the paper.

ESTABLISHED/LOYAL PATIENTS. These patients are the question marks. The biggest temptation is to take them for granted. They come to the office when they should and follow your advice, but you have no evidence that they actively talk about the practice. In this group there are a few champions you have not identified yet. Your task is to flush them out and begin giving them champion acknowledgments. It may take time with some of these stalwarts, and you may not find any champions. Here are a few ideas to help move the champions to the surface and give extra care to the whole group.

1. <u>Private financial consultation is a great benefit to your patients.</u>
Talking with patients about their financial obligations in private will allow you to find out if they are champions. Don't make them stand at a counter and discuss their financial situation where employees or

other patients can hear. If space is at a premium, put up a partition which will block the view of others.

2. Seek their complaints. You will hardly ever hear a word of complaint from loyal patients. Go after the complaints in a positive manner and reward patients when they tell you how your service could be improved.

3. Ask for referrals. It's okay to ask for referrals. You may get some from unlikely sources. When a patient comes through with a referral, give him or her a champion patient reward.

4. Survey your services and recommend additional services. All doctors have a standard set of screening and diagnostic services that they recommend for each type of patient. Men of a certain age need annual colon rectal cancer screening and also may need fitness evaluations and health counseling on other issues. Women who need Pap smears also have other health requirements. Note which patients have health problems that their family members are also likely to have. This is not only good medicine, it is good business. Audit your self-referral protocols and identify areas where you can expand this service to enhance your patients' health. Most of them will appreciate it and feel glad that you took the time to be thorough. The same applies for any new service you start which very few patients have taken advantage of yet. You or the office nurse can develop a very short verbal suggestion that the patient should have the new service performed, stating the reasons why. Patients have the right to decline the offer, but even if they do, they will appreciate the fact that you care about them.

5. Find out if you are getting only one person from the family. Ask the patient where the other significant family members have their healthcare needs taken care of. Before you find out whether the spouse or children have another doctor, let the patient know you would consider it a privilege to serve them as well. If the patient tells you they go to another doctor, no problem. Just let the patient know you will be happy to help if the situation comes up and they need a second opinion or have a medical question. If the other

family members do not have a doctor, you can offer them a discounted service.

6. Network with companies through your patients. An audit of your charts will tell you which companies are represented among your patients. You can simply ask your regular, loyal patients if they know others at work who need a physician (for example, people new on the job who have just moved in from out of town). Have the manager ask how you might attract more employees at the same company. Let patients offer to tell others personally or put up their own personal notes on the company bulletin board telling about your services and their experiences. If they offer to do this, support their efforts with business cards, practice brochures, and a special discount for the first visit or exam. When they respond with referrals, reward them as you would reward your opinion leaders.

OPINION LEADERS/CHAMPION PATIENTS. I've already said a lot about what to do with opinion leaders/champions, but there are many more things you can do. This is a category of patient which cuts across all the other categories. Champions can surface from the ranks of new patients quickly. If new patients meet the criteria for an opinion leader, don't wait for them to go through the normal stages of becoming an established patient before enlisting them to talk for you. Why wait? Study the opinion leader criteria again and keep on the lookout for these types of people. When one comes in, go into action. Champion patients can take time to develop, mostly because it takes time to identify them as opinion leaders. They can also be patients who have been with the practice for a long time and who would die before changing doctors. They know a lot about the practice simply because they have been around a long time. They have settled into a routine of visiting only one doctor and one dentist, and that's it. They have entrusted their healthcare to you for many years and are probably proud of you. These longterm champions believe in you so much that they want you to succeed as if you were family. They not only talk about you to others, they promote you and become your advocates when they hear negative word-of-mouth.

Here are some ideas which will get opinion leader/champion patients talking enthusiastically about your work:

1. Keep them informed. When you have to be in surgery or out on an extended visit, don't just have the receptionist announce that the doctor will be late (many offices don't even do this much). The manager should go into the reception room to inform the waiting patients where the doctor is or call a patient into the room where the receptionist is, give the information personally and then offer the patient a drink (if medically appropriate) or a copy of a new magazine to compensate for the inconvenience. Let the patient keep the magazine. If you are very late, have the staff keep the patient informed and offer to reschedule the visit. Offer your telephone to make local calls for child care arrangements or inform a spouse or work associates. If the wait is at the end of the day, consider giving a gift certificate for lunch or dinner to valuable champion patients as a way to make up for the inconvenience. Your champions will enthusiastically support you if you respect their honor, time, and money.

2. Keep close to them. Pay attention to your patients' needs and let them know you appreciate their support of the practice. Communication is the key for opinion leaders. If they get a couple of extra minutes with you to talk about whatever is on their minds, they will appreciate it. If they see that you are really listening to them, they will be pleased. The doctor is an important person in their lives. They look up to you as an authority figure. It means a lot when you pay attention to them. Speak to them by name often and let them know how much you appreciate their referrals.

3. Acknowledge their written thank you notes. On one wall of the reception room or on one wall in each exam/treatment room post the thank you notes you get from champion patients. You can place the original notes (under glass) on the wall if there is nothing personal about the patient which no one else should see or you can transcribe the notes so that they are more easily read. Typing the notes gives you a chance to edit out personal information which should be kept confidential. If you choose the latter method, place a notice in small print that the original notes are kept on file in the doctor's office. Call it the wall of champions or the wall of fame to draw attention to it. A

subheading can explain that these notes are from valued patients who thought highly enough about the practice to refer their friends and families. In this case you are not the champion or the famous one. You are drawing attention to the patients by acknowledging their contributions to your practice through word-of-mouth. The notes can be about you or about your staff or the whole office. Don't have any thank you notes? The office nurse can ask for a few notes from valued champion patients. He or she can tell them that the staff members are doing a special recognition for the doctor and want several thank you notes from patients to present to the doctor at a special lunch meeting. Tell them that the staff may post the notes in the reception room for all to see. Have the staff give them note paper and a pen to use right in the office.

Why will a wall of fame work? It gives champion patients great pride to see their thank you notes acknowledged and valued. It gives them something else to talk about to their friends. It is a momentous testimony for new patients who are in the reception room or treatment room waiting for the doctor. Here you are using written word-of-mouth marketing for all your patients. Don't want to post the notes on the wall for some reason? No problem. Just put the notes in a big three-ringed notebook titled *Our Patient Hall of Fame* and let it sit with the magazines in the reception room. The first page of the book should be a personal letter from the doctor explaining how valuable these patients are to the practice and noting that they think highly enough of the practice to say so and refer their friends and family members.

4. Guarantee your service. Only recently has the medical practice management literature spoken about making guarantees. If you guarantee that champion patients will never have to wait more than thirty minutes to see you and that you back the offer up with your dollars, you will have enthusiastic patients who will brag about the practice to others. So what if a few new patients come into the practice because they want the same guarantee? Isn't that the point? You must be prepared to back up your guarantee with money to make it right for the patient. There are a lot of things you can do to make it right, such as offering the visit at half price, or offering tickets for two for lunch,

offering two theater tickets, a magazine subscription, or something else of value. Above all, don't keep the guarantee a secret, hoping no one will cash in on it. Instead, make an important event out of it by promoting it to your champions. Then follow through when you need to.

5. Find something extra to do on each visit. Here is another great idea to keep champion patients talking about how much they appreciate your practice. Have a cabinet in the office designated as the champion cabinet; it should contain a videotape lending library, a magazine cache, or a collection of health and beauty aid products or leisure-time products. You may wish to adjust the contents of the cabinet seasonally to reflect the changing needs of patients. In the summer months you can have two or three starter kits for a family barbecue or back-to-school kits to give children in August, before they shop for school supplies. This is just a starter list. You can get products from pharmaceutical supply companies, durable medical equipment companies, and the like.

6. Make personal phone calls when least expected to overwhelm your champion patients and communicate to them that they are highly valued. When you have a written list of champion patients, you can quickly divide the list on a weekly basis and call a few patients each week. The phone call can be about their health, can be a reminder concerning your medical advice, or can be something important in their lives (graduation, anniversary, birthday, wedding, birth, career accomplishment, referral of a new patient). It can also be a very short call to let them know you appreciate their support of the practice.

7. Find some nonmedical services to offer to champion patients. Nonmedical services? That's right. This is not a new concept to practices that have a clientele they value highly. Look at these ideas for starters:

a. Offer child care for patients twice a week for a few hours a day. Over a year's time this could cost a few thousand dollars, but think of the help it would be for mothers who have small children and need to come in for a yearly physical or Pap smear. Train your child care provider to tell or read the children a story or two every hour. Install a video game or have a few picture books and other toys available.

b. Offer a few social services for geriatric champions, such as helping them and their children find independent living arrangements at the right time or helping them link up with senior visitation programs and other services which keep them active in the community and prevent them from becoming institutionalized prematurely.

c. Offer a one-time support group for special categories of champion patients. Gather a small group of diabetic, low back pain, or hypertensive patients for an informal meeting to discuss their common problems and solutions. Tell them that you do not intend to make a long-term program of it but that if they feel comfortable with each other, they can maintain any level of contact they wish. Have just one or two sessions with them, giving medical and social information and letting them talk and get acquainted. Be sure to take the opportunity to thank them formally for being your patients. Have them invite friends who have similar problems.

8. Ask for referrals if you want to. These champions will gladly respond because they know you appreciate them. Many healthcare practices could grow if the doctor would simply ask for referrals from patients who are talkers. When you ask for referrals, you do not need to provide an incentive. For example, you could surprise a champion patient who refers another opinion leader who then becomes established as a patient by giving a gift certificate for dinner for two or theater tickets for two. Acknowledging and saying thank you for a referral after it has happened are important.

9. If you make a mistake in billing, correct it immediately. Don't say, "I'll look into the matter and talk with the manager tomorrow," unless you really cannot resolve the matter without that person. Loyal patients are not out to rip you off. They may sometimes misunderstand a billing, or you may make an error. No problem. Just correct it quickly. The faster you give the solution, the more likely it is that they will be overwhelmed with gratitude and will talk about it with someone else.

10. Provide just-in-time service. This will bond patients to you, and they will talk about it to their friends at work. Here is how this works. Every time you have a champion patient scheduled to come into the office, have his or her name marked with a star or another symbol to alert the receptionist. At just the right time before the appointment, have the receptionist call to give the patient an up-date of how close the office is to being on schedule. If you are running fifteen minutes late, let them know. If you are an hour late because of an emergency, let them know ahead of time so they can adjust their work or errands to meet the change. They will love you if they can get extra work done before coming to the office. You will want to let them know that you will be calling them to tell them how close to schedule you are on the appointment day. Find out what phone number to use (home, work, etc.). If they will not be at a phone, encourage them to call you about half an hour in advance of the appointment time to check.

Note: You may be thinking that this is a lot to offer, that it will take someone a lot of time to coordinate, and that some of your other patients may come to expect this type of service. Never in this material have I promised a quick way to conduct word-of-mouth marketing. Yes, it does take someone's time and commitment to make it happen. However, the payoff is usually far superior to what you can get with any other method.

11. Make your statements of gratitude and acknowledgments for referrals personal. You do this by focusing on your own feelings, such as feeling honored, inspired, elated, grateful, delighted, enthusiastic, confident, eager, expectant, contented, and proud. Don't use a generic phrase like "I feel good about having you as a patient." This is overused and communicates nothing. Be specific about your feelings, let your face show the feeling, and the patient will get the message loud and clear.

NONPATIENT OPINION LEADERS/CHAMPIONS. There are a variety of people who have contact with you and a host of potential patients. This could be the senior citizen transportation service, the taxi driver, the pharmacist, the social worker, the head nurse at the extended care facility, professional conservator, or a host of others. This group can be mined for referrals by using the following process:

1. Get to know these potential referral sources by name.

2. Evaluate whether you want to be associated with them by referral. Ask yourself: Would I want my patients patronizing this business?

3. Ask them for referrals and offer to refer to them if they are in business.

4. Reward them verbally and in writing when they make a referral. If they are in business, reward them by referring someone to them.

Consider the following:

1. Your staff is linked to several hundred people who you don't even know yet. If they see how much you care for your patients, they will become willing referral sources. They see what goes on behind the scenes when patients are not around. If you model ethical behavior during the private times, they will refer their friends and families. Ask them about the organizations they belong to and then ask how you can attract patients from those groups or if they can think of a way to spread the word about the practice. If they like what they see in the practice, it is more than likely that they will be willing to make referrals. They may even tell you how they will do it. If they hesitate, they may have seen something they don't like, or perhaps they don't understand the impact your word-of-mouth marketing efforts are having on patients.

2. Non-healthcare business neighbors are also potential sources of referrals. You can develop cross-promotional programs in which you display their business cards prominently if they agree to do the same. Be sure to check out these business owners carefully before suggesting this so that your level of trust and confidence will be high. When you refer someone to their business, let them know who it was and when the referral occurred. If the referral business turns out to be a

one-sided affair with you giving all the referrals, you don't have to continue referring to them.

3. <u>Healthcare professionals can refer to you</u>. Get to know them first and then offer to do cross-promotional efforts (passing out business cards, sharing the costs of coupons for discounted services, etc.). Introduce yourself to receptionists and managers. Have your manager or nurse meet some of these people for lunch. She or he should take along a few resumes and business cards when going to lunch. Creating and maintaining referrals from other health professionals involves getting to know them personally and discussing issues that are important to them (accomplishments, personal battles won, personal avocational interests, etc.). If you value their referrals, do the following on a consistent basis: take them out to eat, be available, respond immediately when they have a professional favor to ask, keep in constant communication on consultations you perform for them, thank them for their referral, and check the results of your marketing program.

Track the results by keeping a small note card in your pocket or a sheet of paper on your desk with the names of referring professionals and the number of referrals per month they send you. With this chart, you can visually check for changes in referral patterns immediately. If you notice referrals dropping off, see them in person immediately to evaluate the situation. Are they simply slow that month, or were they on vacation? Remind them that you are available any time they need help on a case. If you keep in close contact with them, you will know this before they go on vacation and will know why referrals drop off during this time. When you hear they are going on vacation, ask them who is covering for them. Then make contact with the covering physician to let him or her know you regularly take referrals from the vacationing doctor and are glad to help while the doctor is gone.

4. <u>Community service organizations already know you or know the types of people who are your patients (see Chapter 11)</u>. This may be a volunteer organization at a hospital, a social service agency, or a government-sponsored health agency. The key people to know here are the managers and those who actually deal with clients: case

managers, nurses, and administrative assistants for example. These people should have your resume and take the grand tour of the office, meeting all the key employees they will speak to on the telephone when they call you. Make a commitment to promote their organizations among your patients. Offer to give speeches or in-service educational talks to their staffs. Offer to be on the advisory board of one of these groups. Offer to make a donation to the cause. If you do any of these things, they will love you and become champions for you.

CONCLUSION

Not all these tactics will apply equally well to your practice. Pick those activities which seem to fit most naturally. Adjust them for your style and philosophy and stick to them consistently. The most important thing to remember is to do something and do it on a consistent basis. If you are a bit overwhelmed with how much can be done, remember that these are just ideas. What counts is putting them into action.

Chapter 5

Stopping Negative Word-of-Mouth

To be truly helpful, a book like this must cover the dark side of grapevine marketing. If you spend most of your marketing resources promoting positive word-of-mouth marketing without addressing the problems, you will simply bring in a lot of patients who will become angry and will tell a lot of other people about it. This is one of the best ways to bring an agonizing end to a medical practice. Most medical practices do not die sudden deaths, however. It is the slowly growing negative word-of-mouth dynamic which is the most difficult to detect and treat.

I have been a member of customer service solution teams and have observed that stopping negative word-of-mouth requires that management personnel get specific about problems and solutions. Encourage your patients to be specific when they have complaints. Only with the details in hand can you address the problem and find a solution. If you focus on the details of what actually happened, you can avoid a witch-hunt or a rogue's gallery experience for your staff.

ARE COMPLAINERS ALLIES OR PESTS?

Certain types of patients flit from doctor to doctor, refusing to follow medical advice while they are finding fault with each office. No matter what you do, they will find fault. This type of pathological complainer is not the focus of this book. I don't have any creative solutions for dealing with these patients except to say that you can cut your losses by graciously yet formally cutting them loose from the professional-patient relationship. You will waste a lot of money and time trying to solve their problems when you could be addressing a host of champion patients who could be making referrals to you.

Let us consider the rest of your clientele. Do you hear yourself or your coworkers talking about some of your patients as "pests" or "problems" who take you away from more important work? You may have already guessed where I'm going with this. My biases show.

In the final analysis, patients are your economic bread and butter. Your career exists because of patients. The majority are kind-hearted and good-natured and would not wish you harm under normal circumstances. In fact, most are willing to help you with information which will help you serve them better. In a word, patients are your best allies as well as your best marketing resource. If you catch yourself thinking about a patient as a pest, ask yourself the following questions:

1. Why is this patient so upset? Is there something else going on here that I don't understand? Have I said or done something which made matters worse? Is something happening in a patient's life which is totally unrelated to the visit to the office?

2. Why is the patient continuing to rub my nose in the problem now that I have offered a solution? Does the patient think I do not understand his or her true feelings?

3. If this patient leaves the office in a wrought-up emotional state, what negative word-of-mouth will result? Does this person have an extensive social network? Is this patient a natural opinion leader to whom others look for advice on healthcare? If not, is the patient a family member of an opinion leader?

4. Why don't I see this patient as an ally to help office improve the quality of service? What emotional baggage am I carrying around which is preventing me from seeing this patient as an ally? Why am I feeling inconvenienced and pestered by this patient now?

AVOID ISOLATION

The worst thing that can be done in trying to stop negative word-of-mouth is to act as if it didn't exist. The next worst thing is to belittle the importance negative word-of-mouth has for a medical practice. Cloistering yourself in the office will only reinforce whatever negative feelings the patient has. A subtle form of isolation occurs when the doctor listens to a patient who has a complaint, promises to get back to the patient soon, and drops the issue once the patient leaves. Isolation is a default solution to negative word-of-mouth; it only compounds the problem.

IMPLEMENT A COMPLAINT-GATHERING PROGRAM

I recommend actively looking for problems to correct. Here's why:

1. If you don't know the specific problems patients experience, how will you be able to fix them?

2. If you are not talking to your patients in a way that allows them to be open with you, how will you be able to meet their changing needs?

3. Patients who have a chance to talk with you about a problem, are much more likely to remain loyal in spite of the problem.

Your complaint-gathering program is your way of taking the pulse of the patient community. Without such listening, your office can lose touch with reality very quickly. Remember that only a minuscule portion of your patients will offer to tell you when they are upset, irritated, disappointed, frustrated, or angry. You have to look for problem areas if you expect to get answers.

Complaint-gathering programs come in a variety of forms. It doesn't matter which approach you select as long as you are consistent and the method you choose fits naturally with your approach to healthcare. What is important is that you doggedly follow one method. Here are some examples of how complaints can be gathered without causing more problems among your patients:

Telephone exit interviews

Direct mail surveys

In-office suggestion boxes (survey)

Personal in-office exit interview

Impromptu interviews

1. Use the telephone to call patients the day or evening after an office visit. Ask them if they found the service satisfactory? Was there anything you should know about the visit that will make future visits better? Were they treated courteously by all the staff members? Were they able to get an appointment when they wanted it? Did you spend enough time with them? Did they think you and the staff were competent? Did anything they experienced leave them uncomfortable or uneasy? Asking these types of questions on the telephone will cost you more than using any other method, as you or someone in the office can easily spend five to ten minutes with each patient. If this is too costly, you could pick patients at random or call just the champion patients or the patients who seemed to be the most concerned during a visit. If you use the telephone, you will be able to gather much more information than is possible with any other means. You may even be able to identify specific problems which can be solved quickly.

2. Use direct mail to survey patients one or two days after a visit. Before patients leave the office, tell them they will receive a short survey in the mail. Ask for a commitment to complete it and send it back. Make sure the survey form is easy to complete. Also, include a postage-paid envelope for returning the form. You will get a slightly lower level of response with this method, but it will cost much less than a telephone program. A variation on this is to distribute the survey forms and postage-paid envelopes when patients exit the office and then ask for their commitment to complete the survey form and mail it back within twenty-four hours.

3. Placing suggestion boxes in each exam room or in the reception room is another way to gather helpful information. If you use the

suggestion box, do not make it a passive system. You can have a small poster by the suggestion box explaining why it is there, but you need to personally inform all your patients what the suggestion box is for and ask for a commitment to complete the short card before they leave the office. Tell them that you take suggestions seriously and that their opinions and feedback will help you improve their experience and the experiences of those whom they refer to the office.

4. An exit interview is another useful method for gathering information. This is similar to the telephone call in regard to the amount of time you will have to spend. It also gives you more information than paper and pencil surveys. The exit interview is conducted by the manager or head nurse just before the patient leaves. Use a few prepared questions similar to those suggested above for telephone interviews. Explain why you do exit interviews and state that you value their suggestions for improving your service.

5. Use an impromptu interview with a patient who seems upset in the office. If you notice nonverbal indicators that a patient is irritated, anxious, frustrated, angry, or disappointed, take the patient into a private room for a discussion. Here are some of the nonverbal flags to watch for:

Facial expressions

Tone of voice

Aggressive actions

Here are some opening questions you can use to solicit feedback:
   "I was noticing you here today, and I'm wondering if there is anything I need to know that will help us serve you better."
   "I want to make sure we do all we can to make your experience with us a positive one. Is there something I can do to make your visit better today?"
   "You seemed upset a few minutes ago. Is there something I can do to help make your visit more pleasant?"
   "You seemed so happy when you first came in today. Is there something we have done to change that?"
   Avoid asking "Is everything okay?" since most people will simply

say yes and drop the matter quickly. That approach gets you nowhere if you are certain that the person is in fact upset about something. After you have stated that you are interested in a problem, if the patient refuses to tell you what is wrong, don't push the patient into a corner. Just say, "If you ever need to tell me something that will make your visit here more pleasant, I will be happy to talk with you."

It does not matter which type of complaint-gathering system you use as long as you use it consistently and openly with the patients. The patients must know what types of information you are gathering and why the information is important to you. You can openly link the surveys with the fact that you know they can refer other people to your office. They also have a choice in regard to returning to your office rather than going elsewhere. You value their patronage and want the relationship to continue.

Now that you have specific suggestions for improving patient services, what are you going to do about it? Here's what I suggest to enhance accountability and responsiveness:

1. Log all complaints, using a written description of who is involved on both sides of the issue.

2. Categorize the complaints into natural groupings.

3. Include a place in the log for information such as who the complaint is assigned to for follow-up, the type of solution chosen, and the results perceived by the patient.

4. At the monthly staff meeting, set aside time to identify new problems, solutions to unresolved problems, and the results of solved problems.

ESTABLISH AN "INSTANT SOLUTION" PROGRAM

The faster you can respond to a patient's problem, the more likely that patient will not even remember that there was a problem. The slower you are in responding, the more likely it is that the problem will become significant. Think about it from a patient's point of view. If you have experienced awful service and have screwed up the courage to confront the office about the problem, the last thing you want is to be told to wait for someone else to handle the problem. To an upset patient, waiting is like a punishment for raising the complaint in the first place. The key is *speed*.

Most organizations are geared for a slow, methodical approach to solving consumer's problems. There are formal procedures which must be followed, including specific people who must give approval first, time to research the options, time to confirm the details of the problem, time to analyze which part of the complaint is fact and which part is fiction, an office discussion about the patient and the patient's "true" motives, and a careful rechecking of office policies to make sure you are not giving away the store. I'm not suggesting that rules and formal policies be thrown out; I'm merely saying that a patient's complaints should be addressed quickly. If you act instantly to solve the problem, you risk nothing, but you gain respect from the patient, avert a potential word-of-mouth disaster, and walk away from the situation knowing you did your best.

Here's how an instant solution program works. It must be followed by you as well as every office employee who may hear a complaint. When a patient brings a complaint to you, move to a private room immediately. This will help the patient relax and will communicate to the patient that you are interested in what he or she has to say. Answering the telephone in the middle of hearing a complaint will raise the patient's level of discontent. Having employees walk in with questions unrelated to the problem will make the patient even angrier. Patients want to be heard. If you give them that, they immediately begin to relax even if it doesn't show at first. Do not tell a patient "My nurse will take care of it for you." Instead, call the office nurse into the private room immediately. Explain in your own words what you understand the problem to be and say that you want to correct it. Then tell the patient that while you are serving another patient, the nurse will take the next step and that if the patient has any further questions, he or she should feel free to speak with you again about it.

If a member of the staff first receives the report of a problem, that person should have the authority to implement a solution immediately. If the staff member has to check with you before resolving the matter, speed is of the essence. If you are in the middle of performing a history and physical examination or a complex procedure, a patient with a complaint may have to wait a few minutes. In this case the staff should explain the specific reason for the delay and find out whether it is acceptable to the patient to wait.

Next, surprise the patient by acknowledging the mistake and owning up to it openly. Most consumers are used to getting a runaround. Instead, say, "I'm sorry you experienced this problem. I take full responsibility for what you experienced. I appreciate your bringing this to my attention so we can do something about it quickly. Thank you for bringing this to my attention." If you try to duck the problem by suggesting that someone else in the office probably made the mistake, the patient will feel that you are not interested. Finding fault will not get you to a solution. What works is to quickly acknowledge what patients say as true because for them it is true.

The next step is just as surprising to most people. Before an angry patient can catch his or her breath, state to the patient that you have been given the authority to make it up in some way right now. In consideration for the fact that the patient has had this problem, you are prepared to offer a discount on the visit, or will give the patient a health video or a copy of a health magazine to take home and enjoy. Before you make a specific offer, ask what the patient would like to see happen to rectify the situation. "What can I do to make it right for you right now?" (Note the continued emphasis here on an instant solution.) The patient may merely want to vent anger and leave with the sense that he or she was heard. Or the patient may want some financial consideration.

If the patient says that he or she only wanted to let you know about the problem and needs nothing further, thank the patient sincerely and then offer something in gratitude for telling you about the problem (a free magazine, a health video, or something else of tangible value that confirms the importance of the complaint). You may think this is not necessary. You may be right, but why not send the patient out of the office satisfied, happy, and surprised? You will create positive word-of-mouth about your responsiveness.

If the patient asks for something reasonable, accept it immediately. (This requires that you have had some planning sessions to study the limits of what you can give in consideration.) If such patient's are not sure what they want, make an offer like "Would taking half off your out-of-pocket expenses for today's visit be a fair way to settle it for you?" It may be nice to promise that during the next visit you will work such patients in immediately when they arrive so they will not have to wait. A promise of excellent service in the future is not, however, the solution to today's problem.

Note: The longer you wait to get to this point, the more the patient will want in consideration. The more quickly you can settle on something fair, the less you will spend in the long run.

Finally, reinforce the fact that the patient brought this problem to your attention. This is a great opportunity to tell the patients that you value their trust and appreciate their patronage.

Implementing an instant solution program will cost money once in a while. But think of the damage one person can do by spreading negative word-of-mouth about how unresponsive your office is and saying that you don't care about your patients. Besides, you can set limits on what the employees may and may not offer as an instant solution so they do not offer each complainer the moon. (Some offices may authorize an employee to spend up to $25 or the equivalent of half off a regular office visit.)

HEADING OFF PROBLEMS BEFORE THEY BEGIN

Prevention is the best cure for word-of-mouth problems, but it is human nature to wait until there is a problem before doing something about it. I can hear the logic wheels turning. If something is not a known problem to patients, why change it? Changing something that was not a problem may create a problem you didn't count on. To these and the other reasons we normally give for not fixing problems before they surface, I answer:

1. It may not seem like a problem yet simply because the patients have not said anything about it. But they could be experiencing irritation, frustration, or confusion because of problems in the office. What do you think would happen if you removed these thorny irritations? Would they complain if you made their lives easier? I doubt it. They will probably remark about it the next time you saw them. And they will probably say something about it the next time a conversation swing takes them in that direction when they talk with a friend. Fixing a problem may be just the thing to start them talking about your office to others.

2. Perhaps patients think that the problem is simply the way things are supposed to be in a doctor's office. Their expectations so completely engulf the problem that it has never dawned on them that things could be different. Should you count your blessings? Not necessarily. Your goal is to bring patients back and get them to bring in their friends and families. You may be able to do this by making things different from what they are used to at other offices.

3. It's more convenient to wait until a problem shows up before you do something about it. But when the problem presents itself, you have to spend more energy taking care of it because you not only are taking care of the problem and fixing it for the future, you also have to take care of the negative feelings of the patient. This doesn't seem very efficient to me: it seems like a waste of valuable time and money.

Here are some examples of heading off problems before they loom up and bite you.

1. When you refer a patient to another provider such as a specialist or a hospital, follow up with both the specialist and the patient to confirm that the patient got there. Did the patient receive the kind of care you had planned? This not only creates an opportunity to prevent misunderstandings, it also clearly communicates to patients that you want things to go smoothly. It's okay to check up on the hospital or specialist and help them with word-of-mouth marketing: this can only help you. Ask your patients if there is anything they need help with understanding or doing until they see you again. If you treat referral organizations as an extension of your office in regard to customer service, you will

have happier patients because they will have fewer encounters with other people's mistakes. Does it cost you? Yes. Is it worth it? Yes. I know some people think it's not their job to improve the customer service of the organizations to whom they send patients, but if you don't help, it could eventually reflect negatively on you and your work if something goes wrong. The patient may choose another doctor because of the negative experience with referrals.

2. What if the manager is out of the office when a patient calls with a question or a complaint? What if the only person in the office is the receptionist or the janitor? What are they instructed to do when a patient or a referring doctor with a complaint calls or shows up? I've intentionally called doctors' offices at lunchtime or near closing time to see how the call is handled. You would be surprised at what I get when I call. I'm routinely told by one office, "Can you call back in the afternoon when the manager is supposed to be here?" Another person will simply say, "I don't know. You will have to call back later." No wonder patients get angry. Proper training is the only prevention for this type of word-of-mouth problem.

3. Do you have a foolproof way to transfer information between the various people involved in the patient's care: the hospital, the specialist, the nurse, the doctor, the receptionist, the medical assistant, the manager, and so forth? A small mistake in information transfer can cause great inconvenience for a patient. Create a system of checks and balances to minimize the risk of missing important information. Where is the system breaking down the most? Where are the weak links in the information chain? What can you do to correct it before a public relations nightmare occurs? What you are attempting to do here is plug up the cracks through which things tend to slip at the most crucial time or when least expected.

MAKE CHANGES VISIBLE AND COMMUNICATE

As you implement a problem-seeking program, you are bound to find at least a few things you can do differently to improve patient satisfaction. If a patient puts a good suggestion in the suggestion box, follow through on it. Then communicate to all patients what the suggestion was and what you have done about it. To do this, you may want to put a poster in the reception room. Putting it in each exam room will have more of an impact because patients can focus on just that one message while they are waiting for the doctor. Having a notice in the exam rooms gives the doctor and nurse a chance to speak with each patient personally about the suggestion and what was done. Personal, face-to-face conversations are much more powerful, especially if you use these opportunities to suggest to patients that they can refer others to the practice. You can also state that you are open to other suggestions.

Chapter 6

The Cost of Word-of-Mouth

I've already mentioned that word-of-mouth marketing is not free. It costs you something to offer excellent service. It costs to promote a referral-based practice. Therefore, the issue is not whether this type of marketing costs you, it is whether it costs more not to have a word-of-mouth marketing program than to have one. It is a matter of determining whether word-of-mouth marketing costs more than other promotional methods for the same return.

I'm making three claims here that are consistent with the direction of the whole book:

1. Positive word-of-mouth marketing will cost less cash and will bring a larger return on investment than will most other promotion methods. Do more of the positive.

2. Negative word-of-mouth will cause a loss of potential revenue and probably some cash. It can easily cancel out positive word-of-mouth marketing. Try to stop the negative.

3. Without a word-of-mouth marketing program which addresses both the negative and positive dynamics, your other promotional efforts will probably cost more money.

Here's what I mean.

First, positive word-of-mouth marketing costs less than other forms of promotion. Where else can you get patients just by asking for them? Asking for a referral costs nothing, but when you ask a satisfied patient to refer someone else, you are getting something almost for nothing. You can't beat that. Even if you decide to spend a little cash to show appreciation, you can spend it after the referral has brought you revenue, so you're still not out anything. Where else can you spend your marketing dollars after the promotion has done its work? Every other form of promotion requires that you spend and risk money before a return is guaranteed. This is not the case with word-of-mouth marketing. The obvious exception to this is the staff labor which is expended in the course of providing excellent service.

Second, positive word-of-mouth marketing traditionally produces a better return on your promotional investment. If you spent $5,000 on a yearlong marketing campaign, what financial return would you get? I did some research recently in a southern California city, and here's what I found as I compared several different promotional tactics. (I realize that not all geographic areas are the same.)

1. Yellow Pages: For $5,000 you could get about a fifth of a page (one color) plus two column listings. The response will vary by specialty and how much consumer demand exists for certain services. You could get from just one or two new patients a month up to five or ten. Track the results carefully. Some practices get 10 or even 15 percent of all their new patients from the Yellow Pages, but don't assume that you will. One doctor did a test of his Yellow Pages advertising to check how many calls he got. He purchased a separate phone line with a previously unpublished number. He advertised the new number in one Yellow Pages book only. The result: he averaged about thirty calls a month on the new phone line. This didn't translate into thirty new patients each month, however. Some of his own patients had to look up his number in the Yellow Pages. Some of the callers had the wrong number. A few were interested in the doctor's services. A few became new patients. You have to be in the book, but do you have to spend $5,000 to get good marketing results? The sad thing is that if you triple or quadruple this type of advertising, you may not get much better results. Another factor is that you could be in two or more competing telephone books concurrently. Please don't misunderstand my intentions here: I'm not out to bash the Yellow Pages. But compared with what you can get from word-of-mouth marketing, the Yellow Pages book pales into insignificance.

2. Newspaper: For $5,000 you can get a fourth of a page in the local daily paper six times a year or a fourth of a page in a weekly paper a

dozen or so times a year. To be effective, most medical services must include a special offer, a free test, a free public education event, or something which will attract patients' interest. The response could be up to 50 to 100 new people who want the special offer. As many as a fourth of these individuals may "convert" into patients if they are not part of an HMO or the established patients of another doctor. But long-term results are questionable for most specialties. I've seen office administrators throw thousands of dollars at newspaper advertising when following the well-meaning counsel of a marketing consultant. This reminds me of the saying "I know I just wasted half of my advertising budget, but I don't know which half."

3. <u>Practice Brochure</u>: The practice brochure is the most misunderstood marketing tactic. Many physicians believe they need one but don't know how to use it. A practice brochure can be helpful in a word-of-mouth marketing program, can sit on a shelf, or can be used without purpose. By itself, it represents a large marketing expenditure. You may decide that you need a brochure to give to your champion patients or to leave behind after giving community speeches. For now, just consider the cost compared with the low-cost word-of-mouth marketing tactics you can use without a practice brochure. Including graphic art, copywriting, photos, and two-color printing, you can easily spend over $5,000 to get 3,500 or 4,000 copies. The results you get depend on how you use it. The response to this vehicle by itself will be minimal if any. This one is difficult to track for results unless you put a special offer in the brochure and distribute it to new people. Used this way, it is a real crap shoot. When you use a modest brochure or a doctor's resume (at a much lower cost) in conjunction with your word-of-mouth marketing program, you are carefully targeting the brochure at specific people who are likely to give it to someone who is looking for a doctor. However, word-of-mouth marketing can function quite well without a brochure because the strength of the program lies not in the printed page but in the power of the personal verbal communication given by a satisfied patient.

4. <u>Direct Delivery</u>: For $5,000 you can have professionally printed "door hangers" delivered five times a year to 8,000 households. I've tried this type of promotional tactic. It works better for some types of

medical practices, especially urgent care centers, to target "unattached" patients, areas that are not heavily saturated with managed care plans, or crisis intervention patients. The responses will be for a special offer such as deeply discounted blood tests or exams. The long-term results may be poor if you get a 1 percent response and a fourth of those individuals "convert" into permanent patients. If you're lucky, you may get fifty new people who want to be patients, and not all of them will have commercial insurance. My only comment here is that this isn't pizza we are selling. I am a firm believer in direct marketing, but a one-time burst into a neighborhood with direct delivery doesn't compare with a long-term consistently applied internal marketing program that develops word-of-mouth.

5. Word-of-Mouth: Take 100 champion patients and spend up to $50 on them during the year to acknowledge their support of your reputation and give them superior service. Overwhelm them with excellent service the two, three, or four new patients they bring in. You will end up with 200, 300, or even 400 happy new patients, many of whom will become loyal referral sources in the future. Don't scoff at these numbers, for they are entirely possible to achieve in markets not heavily saturated by managed care. Big returns are possible even in heavy managed care markets. One of the advantages of this type of promotion is that you don't often need to spend $50 on each champion patient to get this kind of return on your investment. Besides all these new patients, you also get a much more smoothly running service system, motivated employees, and the sense of accomplishment which comes only from developing a word-of-mouth practice.

RETURN ON INVESTMENT

In several places I have mentioned this financial term as if it were a magical litmus test for marketing. I've also made the claim that word-of-mouth marketing will produce much higher rates of return on a promotional investment. Even if this is true, what does it mean? Some marketing consultants will tell you that a ten to one return on investment gives you ten dollars of gross revenue for every dollar you spend on promotion. Here's an example.

Suppose you spent $1,000 on a promotional program to build business volume. With a tracking system in place, you can confirm that you bring in fifty new patient visits, each bringing an average of $100 per visit. Using the above method, you can calculate the return on investment (ROI) at five to one. An ROI of five to one would constitute dramatic results from any type of medical promotion.

This is a rather crude way of reckoning ROI, but some find it useful. I prefer to include in the formula a factor for what it costs you to perform the service during the 50 new patient visits (in other words, basing ROI on an estimated *net* pretax revenue rather than on gross revenue).

With my personal addition to the formula, the return drops to a low level. Using the same example and subtracting 50 percent for the expenses involved in performing the service, your return on investment will be 2.5 to 1. Whether you choose my method or the simpler version, stick to it to compare one promotional method with another. Be sure to track the results.

One of the difficulties in word-of-mouth marketing is achieving a consistent implementation of the principles. What may appear to be a low return on your investment may simply indicate a problem with implementation.

THE COSTS OF NEGATIVE WORD-OF-MOUTH

This is where you probably expect me to bring down the hammer on negative word-of-mouth. I won't disappoint you because it helps make the point about how important a positive word-of-mouth marketing program is.

There are three sources of cost when negative word-of-mouth occurs:

1. The first source of "lost revenue" occurs when unhappy patients decide to go to another doctor. You could argue that this doesn't really cost cash out of your pocket, and I would grant you this much. However, if these patients had remained satisfied in your care, all things being equal, they would have returned to you for care and you would have made more money. As was noted before, as many as 30 or 40 percent of patients are dissatisfied enough to leave a practice in favor of another doctor, while up to 60 percent contemplate switching to a new doctor. If each patient represents four office visits a year, you could lose about a fourth of this without instituting a word-of-mouth marketing program. The insidious thing about this type of lost revenue is that it happens very slowly. You don't wake up some morning and suddenly realize that you are $75,000 poorer because of negative word-of-mouth.

2. Another source of "cost" is what it costs to replace dissatisfied patients who take their money elsewhere. In most businesses the rule of thumb is that it costs a business as much as five times more to garner a new consumer than it costs to keep a happy consumer coming back. In a positive word-of-mouth marketing program it may not cost you this much. It all depends on how good your champions are in bringing new patients who will stay with the practice. If it costs, for example, $8,000 per year in marketing and you have a base of 1,675 patients in the practice, you are spending about $5 per patient on marketing. Remember that it can cost up to five times as much to get new patients. Thus, the true replacement costs for dissatisfied patients can represent cash out of your pocket if you want to maintain the volume you had before losing the unhappy patients. Group practices can monitor the marketing costs of replacing unhappy patients by department or by physician. For example, if the member services department observes that during one quarter of the year twenty patients leave the group because of dissatisfaction with one department or one physician, marketing replacement costs can be estimated. At $25 per lost patient, the estimated replacement cost attributed to the department or physician is $500. Giving departments and physicians this type of information on the economic side of negative word-of-mouth builds awareness about the importance of good service.

3. The third source of "cost" is more difficult to monitor, yet it raises the simple point that if you have a problem with negative word-of-mouth, you are going to miss the opportunity to serve some patients who would have come to you if they had not heard a horror story from dissatisfied patients. Counting actual numbers here is impossible. Because of this, I will leave this source of cost out of the following example.

4. Another source of cost is the amount of staff time that it takes to solve problems, deal with unhappy patients, and the resulting lower productivity.

Tables 6–1 and 6–2 summarize the costs of negative word-of-mouth and the value of positive word-of-mouth. The actual dollar amounts can be adjusted for your situation. Large medical groups will have a more complex revenue picture. Medical groups that are contract providers with health maintenance organizations are potentially even more at risk from negative word-of-mouth. If an office continually makes health plan members angry about poor service, the health plan may remove that office from the provider panel rather than risk losing members. Losing a health plan contract can mean the loss of even the happy patients who are trying their best to extend your positive reputation, something which they may do even after being informed that they may no longer use you as their doctor.

There is no more striking example of negative word-of-mouth than the case of patients who are assigned to a physician in a "capitated" program where the medical group receives a certain amount of money each month for each health plan member. If negative word-of-mouth results in your contract being terminated by the health plan which cannot afford to have negative publicity in the community, you may see a swift drop in cash flow as this capitated payment evaporates. If you have such a sudden decrease in office revenue, some of your personnel may have to be laid off. You may have to do a lot of extra work trying to convince the health plan that grievance procedures were followed precisely. Even after all the time and energy you put into saving your contract with the health plan, you still may lose it.

Word of mouth marketing programs are designed to be imple-

Table 6-1
The Cost of Negative Word-of-Mouth

Revenue From Positive Word-of-Mouth	
None	$0.00
Lost Revenue	
Annual gross revenue	$400,000.00
Patients	1,675
(@ 4 visits/year including in-pt days)	
6700 visits; Length of in-pt stay of 4 days/	
discharge)	
Percentage of patients who leave	18.75%
(assume 25% are dissatisfied and 75% of these	
leave)	
Number of dissatisfied patients who leave	314
Average revenue per patient	$238.80
Lost Revenue	$74,983.20
(314 × $238.80)	
Replacement Costs	
Marketing Costs	$8,000.00
Average cost per patient	$4.77
Marketing costs for 314 lost patients	$1,497.78
Multiplied by a factor of 5 for replacement	$7,488.90
(314 × $4.77 × 5)	
Summary	
Revenue from positive word of mouth	$0.00
Lost Revenue	−$74,983.20
Replacement Costs	−$7,488.90
Total negative results	($82,472.10)
Results over 10 years	($824,721.00)

Table 6-2
The Value of Positive Word-of-Mouth

Revenue From Positive Word-of-Mouth	
Number of people satisfied patients tell	2,010
(assume 30% tell 4 others)	
Number of new patients who come in	201
(assume just 10% respond)	
New revenue from positive word-of-mouth	$49,998.80
(201 × $238.80)	
Lost Revenue	
Annual gross revenue	$400,000.00
Patients	1,675
(© 4 visits/year including in-pt days;	
6700 visits; stay of 4 days/discharge)	
Percentage of dissatisfied patients who leave	2.5%
(assume 5% unhappy and 50% of these leave)	
Number of dissatisfied patients	42
Average revenue per patient per year	$238.80
Revenue lost through negative word of mouth	$10,029.60
(42 × $238.80)	
Replacement Costs	
Marketing costs	$8,000.00
Marketing costs per patient	$4.77
Marketing costs for 42 lost patients	$200.34
Multiplied by 5 for replacement	$1,001.70
(42 × $4.77 × 5)	
Summary	
Revenue from positive word-of-mouth	$49,998.80
Lost revenue	−$10,029.60
Replacement costs	−$1,001.70
Total positive results	$38,967.50
Results over 10 years	$389,675.00

(An annual difference of over $100,000 compared with the cost of negative word-of-mouth.)

mented by the staff in the course of doing business. In larger offices additional staff should not be hired to manage word-of-mouth. In large multispecialty groups, word-of-mouth marketing may be given to the member services department. In this case, the program can be kept simple enough to be managed without additional salary expense.

The costs of adding five minutes to a new patient's first visit or taking a few minutes to talk with champion patients are not figured in the two tables. These and other incidental expenses of operating a positive word-of-mouth program can be estimated only after you have settled on a specific program that meets your needs.

Not included in the tables are other costs involved with the results of negative word of mouth such as; legal fees, office inefficiency, waste, and low productivity.

Now consider this same medical practice after it establishes a word-of-mouth marketing program to address both the negative and the positive. Through a more consistent customer service program, the losses from negative word-of-mouth are minimized although not completely eliminated. The gains from positive word-of-mouth marketing are enhanced through consistent application of the principles outlined in this book.

CONCLUSION

Does it cost money to get patients? Absolutely. Even if you are in a managed care group which negotiates several contracts every year, the marketing effort costs you cash and time. Advertising costs a huge amount of money and word-of-mouth marketing also costs you. The question here is which type of word-of-mouth will cost you the most. The examples in the tables is hypothetical. Your office could be entirely different. You may be more or less successful at reducing the costs of negative word-of-mouth, and at gaining from positive word-of-mouth marketing.

Chapter 7

Train, Train, Train

I'm sure that by now you understand that word-of-mouth marketing requires a continuing commitment to improve your reputation if you expect to get continuing results. It also requires a high degree of involvement from the staff. The only way this commitment can remain effective over time is through continued learning.

Left to itself over time, word-of-mouth marketing will go from good, to adequate, to bad, to worse as a result of deteriorating awareness and skill. Employees will be hired who do not have the level of interpersonal skills you desire. New equipment will be purchased, requiring new skills. The government, other providers, or health plans will require new procedures. Old habits which place your reputation at risk may surface unexpectedly when job stress increases. Without training on these issues, your office will degrade into a state of confusion. A negative reputation will usually follow.

I recently surveyed the successful customer service programs of fifty leading American companies. One of the common threads was the high priority these companies placed on training. Employees at these firms have come to accept that continual training for word-of-mouth marketing is part of what is expected. When the training is effective, employees do their work better, get positive feedback from clients, complain less, and become more enthusiastic about their work. In other words, not only do well-trained employees enhance the company's reputation, they also have higher morale.

Let's assume you have instituted a training program for word-of-mouth marketing based on this book or other materials on patient relations. It's two months now since you got everyone interested in word-of-mouth marketing. You get to work one morning and realize that the old habits are back; you are letting important marketing details slip through the charts. You listen in on a conversation between your employee and a patient, only to hear excuses given instead of solutions. Patients at the reception window begin complaining about mistakes in billing yet you do not see anyone in the billing department actively looking for ways to prevent these problems. You notice that the only follow-up communication your office has with patients occurs when there are problems to solve. Patients leave the office anxious, frustrated, or angry.

It's time for a refresher course for everyone. It's time to build habits that build your reputation, such as the following:

1. Honesty

2. Positive communication with patients between visits

3. Accepting responsibility when mistakes are made and then making things right immediately

4. Including patients in major office transitions

5. Showing gratitude

6. Communicating personally with patients

7. Availability

8. Confusion-free office operations

What should be next on the training course schedule? Here are a few ideas to draw from as you develop an ongoing training program. Some of the ideas may seem out of place in your office environment. In that case, adapt what seems most useful to you and leave the other suggestions for other offices.

The unique aspect of this list is that you do not need to pay an outside consultant to conduct the training. You can do it yourselves: research, organize, present, practice skills, and evaluate outcomes. Think of it as a repeating clinical rotation in patient services that every staff member is expected to participate in, including yourself.

If you believe that training is for your staff members only, since they seem to have most of the problems with patients, your word-of-mouth marketing program will be undermined. The staff members will go home after work and say to their families, "The doctor expects us to go through all these stupid training programs, but he doesn't attend himself. He's the one that really needs the training." However, if you participate in the training with your staff, you

1. Communicate that you take word-of-mouth marketing seriously. This motivates staff members to be serious about learning skills.

2. Tell them that you are not above learning how to improve your skills with patients. This shows them that everyone is expected to participate. It can reduce the risk of complaints by 100 percent.

SIXTEEN HOME-GROWN TRAINING IDEAS

1. Telephone skills. I often hear the telephone answered "Doctor's office" when I call a doctor. It would be nice to know with whom I am speaking. It would be nice to know that the person answering the phone is interested in talking to me instead of acting like I am a pest. The other telephone phrase I hear a lot in the reception room is "What is your problem?" I know the receptionist is trying to be helpful to the doctor and the nurse, but it leaves the caller wondering if he or she has been an inconvenience to the office. You get the idea here even if you don't agree with my examples. Have the staff practice answering the telephone in ways that help patients know who they are speaking with. They should answer the telephone quickly, within three rings. It is important that they identify your office and themselves by name. They should speak distinctly into the telephone even when they are in a hurry to pick up other lines.

2. Use the "telephone tag game" to improve telephone answering skills. In these simple drills, prepare a list of questions or complaints that require the staff to practice positive skills. The more difficult, the better, since the practice will increase the confidence of the staff in solving telephone problems. The questions are written down on small note cards or papers and shuffled. Have everyone playing the game seated in a circle. Deal one card to each staff member and place the remaining cards in a stack facedown on the table. The person to the left of the dealer reads the card to any staff member in the room. That person's task is to think of a positive response immedi-

ately. If he or she cannot think of a positive response, anyone in the room may answer. Then others who have alternative responses are allowed to contribute their ideas. Play passes to the next person to the left and so on until everyone has a chance to both read a card and answer a card. If you want to keep score, develop a simple point system for giving acceptable answers. One round each staff meeting may be sufficient for skill development to reach the level you desire. Here are some ideas as starters for questions or complaints on your cards.

"May I speak with _____ (substitute the name of one of the staff members)?"

(_____ is on her lunch break.)

"How can I get to Dr. _____'s office from my house?

(substitute the name of a doctor's office across town that you rarely refer to for consultations.)

"Why didn't I get my lab results today?"

"Why did the hospital bill me twice for my x-ray?"

"I already paid for my visit when I was in your office. Now I get a bill for the visit. Can you do something about this?"

"I know the doctor is with a patient, but I want to talk to the doctor now."

"Can I change my appointment to come in on Monday evening?"

"I forgot how many times I am supposed to take these pink pills. What do I do?"

"Can you ask the hospital not to charge me so much when I go in for the test? I don't think my insurance will cover the whole thing."

"I don't have any way to get to your office for my appointment. Can you help me find a ride?"

"Tell the doctor that John called."

Listen to the questions you commonly hear on the telephone and write down some of the complaints and questions you hear from your patients. Add these complaints to your playing cards.

Unacceptable responses include phrases such as, "I don't know," "No" (when it begins a sentence), "You have to ask the doctor," "That's not my job," "I just work here; call back in the afternoon," "We don't have that," "The person who knows that isn't here now," "I don't know when he is coming in," "We're not," and "I'm not sure."

3. Who does what here? Try some training for everyone on job descriptions and policies so that no one will ever have to say "I don't know" to a patient again. If you don't have an office policy and procedure manual, develop one immediately and make sure each employee reads and understands every page. It is best to create one inside a three-ring binder so you can make page revisions without revising the whole document. You are probably required by law to have employee health and safety manuals anyway. Think of your policy and procedure manual as a word-of-mouth marketing safety manual.

4. Technical Skill Review (TSR). At each staff meeting take one piece of office equipment and have a five-minute refresher on how it is to be used properly. During the training emphasize the importance of getting it right the first time. Remind the staff members to avoid letting their frustrations show if the equipment doesn't work correctly. Here is a list of equipment to practice using:

Telephone call transfers (many patients become frustrated because they get cut off or their calls are transferred to the wrong extension.)

Computer scheduling

Fax machine

Clinical equipment

Reception room equipment (television, videotape machines, fish tanks, lamps, etc.)

5. Cross-training in job responsibilities. Why is it important for several people to know how to register a patient, answer questions about office policies and procedures, and do other tasks that require patient involvement? You never know when something will go wrong and

the designated answer person will be out of the office while a patient is there. Cross-training decreases office confusion, builds respect between employees, and gives everyone a stake in the outcome.

6. Error-free treasure hunting. This is a fun way to identify areas for improvement in the office. It is a way to raise the awareness of all employees of the procedures most at risk for errors. It is also a way to conduct problem-solving sessions to correct errors in customer service. This training exercise helps get rid of old ways of thinking about things and old ideas such as "Everyone makes mistakes" and "Let someone else take care of it." Combine this with a promotion program telling your patients you want to develop an error-free office. See how they respond to help you.

7. Worst case scenario. I know this sounds negative, but it is a valuable tool when major office disasters occur. If you have not mentally walked through worst case scenarios ahead of time, you and your patients are in for a rude awakening. For example, what will you do when your computer system crashes? Will you be able to answer patient inquiries, schedule patients, send out reminder notices, and continue your word-of-mouth marketing program? Or will you just blame the computer every time a patient calls with a question? What will your office do if there is a major disaster and you have patients in the office? What will you do for your patients? Think about it. What if a violent or verbally abusive patient comes in and disrupts the whole office? What will you do and say? Think about it now. These negative scenarios represent public relations nightmares. Without a disaster plan in place, you are at risk.

8. We do that here? Take a few minutes at a staff meeting to inform all the personnel about all the services you offer. This keeps them from having to say "I don't know" to patients. It also keeps them alert for additional ways to be of service to the patients. If you don't have a written list of all the services you provide, make one and give everybody a copy.

9. Moments of truth or consequences. During a staff meeting, pick a few of the moments of truth from Chapter 8 and ask your staff,

"What are the consequences if our patients are dissatisfied with this moment of truth? How can we improve their satisfaction today?"

10. How to make our problem solving skills faster. Here is an area where you can really overwhelm patients. If you jump on a problem the moment it is brought to you and solve it so fast that the patient's head is swimming, the patient is not likely to remember that there was even a problem. Here is an area for fruitful brainstorming and cross-training involving the whole office. You will want to develop some policies by yourself, but every person connected with the office can get involved. Start with a brainstorming free-for-all in which any suggestion, no matter how crazy, is accepted for consideration. Set a few brainstorming rules such as the following:

   a. No one is allowed to criticize, laugh at, or disagree with any suggestion for at least the first thirty minutes of brainstorming.

   b. Record on paper all ideas presented for use in later discussions.

   c. Allow any suggestion to be made whether it is a statement of a problem or a statement of a solution.

11. The anticipation game. This is where you enlist the support of the staff and patients to look for potential problems and ask "What can go wrong here?" over and over until you find five or six things which need corrections, before they become problems. It is easy to wait for patients to bring you problems, but what if you can find a few yourself? Why wait for patients to tell you? Correct the problems now and have happier patients now.

12. First impressions. Call someone in who has never been to the office and ask that person to book an appointment as a patient. This person is what we call a "mystery shopper" who can tell you his or her first impressions of the office. You will find that you will get much more helpful information from the mystery shopper if you give this person some basic criteria to go on, such as cleanliness, atmosphere, comfort, staff attitudes, and staff responsiveness. I strongly suggest that the mystery patient be presented with a complete bogus diagnosis and go through the whole office experience. Of course, the services received should be free in consideration for the mystery shopper's time and feedback. Invite this person back to an office staff meeting to present

his or her findings. This will make for interesting discussions and successful problem-solving efforts.

13. Common patient frustrations. This is another brainstorming session in which all employees are given a chance to mention the times they have observed patients either verbally or non-verbally venting their frustration. It may help to give an assignment ahead of time to get employees looking for signs of frustration in patients. During the discussion ask the employees to describe specific behaviors they have observed in patients. This is a valuable training tool in itself. This awareness-building session can turn into a problem-solving session too. Remember that feelings are the flags of happy and unhappy customers. Find out what causes their frustrations and make corrections, and you will have happy patients. Find out what makes them happy and satisfied, and you will improve your reputation.

14. Policy and procedure review. This can be hard to do since it may be difficult to see how policies and procedures create unhappy patients. Unfortunately, policies and procedures are the single largest hidden cause of patient dissatisfaction. Without addressing these two areas, you may be only treating the symptoms of dissatisfaction rather than getting to the root of the problem. Whatever you do, don't leave this one out. This should be done at least twice a year during a formal staff meeting. The other option is to review at least one policy page and one procedure page from your policy and procedure manual during every staff meeting. Ask the following questions:

   a. What is working?
   b. What are we doing differently from what we were doing last year?
   c. Where are the red flags that show things are not working as we wish?
   d. What needs improvement so that patients are served better and our reputation is enhanced?

15. Conflict resolution skills. Here is another practical training program where everyone can get involved practicing actual skills such as how to handle an angry patient or an angry coworker. You may want to get some outside help on this one. Call a local university or psycho-

logical group and ask for someone to come at no charge for this type of training.

16<u>Review of word-of-mouth marketing tactics</u>. You cannot repeat this one too often. Staff members need to be reminded of the specific and important reasons why your office is involved with word-of-mouth marketing. The follow-up training can focus on stopping negative word-of-mouth or promoting positive word-of-mouth. Remind the staff members of the specific action steps you use. Get their feedback on how well they think it is working.

Chapter 8

Making Patients into Champions: Ninety-Plus Things That Can Go Right (or Wrong)

Every patient you care for is a potential champion. Some people may not fit the profile of the typical opinion leader as you think of it. However, if these patients have the opportunity to speak about you only one time to just one other person, they fulfill the role of opinion leader for that other person. That one time may be their shining moment as a champion, and it is a moment you cannot afford to overlook. By giving excellent service at each moment of truth, you can make all your patients champions.

Here are some situations and issues where your patients face the moment of truth. Each represents an opportunity to provide excellent service and create a positive reputation. However, each also represents a corresponding risk of creating dissatisfaction if the experience does not meet the patient's expectations.

The following questions are written as if addressed to one of your patients.

BEFORE THE FIRST CONTACT WITH THE DOCTOR

1. Did you have information about how to contact the doctor's office? (phone number, location, hours of availability, etc.)

2. Did the referring person give you adequate information which added to your positive expectations? (information on the background, experience, office hours, location, parking, names of office personnel who can help, etc.)

3. Have you heard about the doctor or the doctor's work from friends, family members, health plan directories, or other professionals? What kind of reputation does the doctor have?

CALLING FOR AN APPOINTMENT

4. Did you have the correct telephone number?

5. Was the phone call answered promptly?

6. Was the phone call answered courteously?

7. Was the telephone operator competent?

8. Were you put on hold? If so, for how long?

9. Was the telephone operator willing to help?

10. Did the person you spoke with understand what you needed?

11. If your call was transferred, did it get transferred to the correct person the first time?

12. Did you hear negative phrases such as "I don't know," "That's not my job," or "You'll have to ask the doctor about that yourself"?

13. If an answering service took the call, did they ask for the pertinent information and give you helpful information?

14. Did you receive a callback soon after the office employees were scheduled to return to the office?

15. How accessible was the appointment time to you? Were the time of day and the day of week convenient?

16. How many days did you have to wait for the appointment?

17. Were you instructed about what to do and what to bring with you on the day of the appointment?

18. Were you told what the information would be needed when you came for the appointment?

19. Were you informed about a cancellation policy?

20. Did the scheduler offer directions on how to get to the office?

21. Were you informed that you should come early to have paper-work completed?

22. Did the office personnel understand why you wanted to see the doctor and what you needed?

GETTING TO THE OFFICE

23. Were the directions correct and written in language you could follow easily?

24. Did you locate the office quickly?

25. Was the office convenient to your home or place of employment?

26. Could you find the front door easily?

27. Was there adequate parking?

28. Did you feel safe parking and walking to the entrance?

REGISTRATION PROCESS

29. Were you greeted within twenty seconds of your arrival?

30. Did the person greeting you introduce himself or herself by name clearly and distinctly? Did that person ask for your name?

31. Were you greeted courteously and warmly?

32. Was the registration staff willing to help?

33. Were you helped with the registration process, or were you left on your own?

34. Was the registration process completed in time for your appointment?

35. Were you informed what to do next, and where to go after completing the registration process?

36. Did you understand the purpose of the forms you were asked to complete?

37. Did the front office staff seem sympathetic?

38. How long did you wait in the reception room?

39. How long did you wait in the examination room?

40. Was the nurse or assistant sympathetic?

41. Was the doctor on time for the appointment?

42. Were you comfortable while you waited?

43. Was the office clean and free of offensive odors?

44. Were the staff members eager to help?

45. Were the staff members concerned about your privacy?

46. Were the staff members sensitive to the inconvenience of your health problem?

47. Were you briefed before your visit with the doctor about what to expect?

48. Were attitudes toward other patients (in person and on the telephone) positive?

49. Did the staff pay attention to your special needs or requirements?

50. Was the registration process completed correctly the first time?

51. Were you spoken to by name by back office personnel?

52. Was the atmosphere of the office calm?

53. Were any delays explained to you in specific terms that made sense?

MEDICAL SERVICE

54. Did the doctor greet you by name?

55. Was the doctor courteous and warm?

56. Did the doctor seem to be in a hurry?

57. Was the procedure longer or shorter than you expected?

58. Did you have enough time with the doctor?

59. Were your personal belongings safe during the procedure?

60. Were you informed about when test results would be presented to you?

61. Were you informed about what to do next?

62. Did the medical equipment appear to function correctly the first time?

63. Was the procedure performed correctly the first time?

64. Were you informed about how long the procedure would take?

65. Were you informed when the visit was completed?

MAKING FINANCIAL ARRANGEMENTS

66. Did you discuss the financial arrangements in private?

67. Did you understand office payment policies and the reasons for those policies?

68. Did you feel like a valued patient during the financial counseling session?

69. Were you informed about the various options for payment?

70. Were your insurance benefits clear to you?

LEAVING THE OFFICE

71. Could you find your car easily?

72. If you left by taxi or public transportation, did someone help you with information or with a telephone call to make the arrangements?

73. What was your overall level of satisfaction with the office services?

74. What was your level of confidence in the services performed?

75. Did you feel safe walking from the office to your car?

76. Did you get done with the appointment when you expected?

FOLLOW-UP TO THE VISIT

77. Were you informed of test results in a timely manner?

78. Did the test results make sense to you?

79. Were you given recommendations about what to do next?

80. Did the staff seem to be concerned about the side effects and results of the procedure?

81. Were you encouraged to follow through on the medical advice given by the physician and nurse?

82. Were you given adequate information about any hospital procedures which were recommended?

83. Did you receive the information you needed to register with the hospital's outpatient services department?

84. Were you addressed by name?

85. Did the staff person introduce himself or herself by name?

86. Was the financial statement correct?

87. Did you receive all the information which was promised to you?

88. Do you feel like a valued patient?

89. Would you recommend the practice to a friend?

90. Do you feel good enough about the service that you would tell someone else how good it was? (Was the service adequate, or was it exceptional?)

91. If you had a complaint, did the first person you talk to have a solution, or did you get bounced from person to person?

92. Did the office staff members seem to be aware of your feelings, or were they out of touch?

93. What were your first impressions?

94. Would you return to this office for follow-up care?

Chapter 9

Word-of-Mouth Marketing in Managed Care Settings

During one of my word-of-mouth marketing training programs an office manager asked, "We are getting a lot of managed care patients assigned to us. When they call for an appointment, they are really angry that they can't choose their own doctors anymore. Our problem is not how to get new patients. My question is, "How we can keep these new patients, who think they have no choice, from leaving the practice?" Upon closer inquiry, I found that not only were the new managed care patients unhappy, many of the well-established fee-for-service patients were unhappy about the service they were getting as well. The challenge this practice faces is to overwhelm these new patients with such good service that they tell their friends how glad they are that they signed up with the health plan.

Is word-of-mouth marketing important in managed care settings? Here are more real-life examples showing why the answer to this question is yes.

An office manager at another seminar told me that her practice was part of an Independent Practice Association, (IPA) and therefore functions as a panel provider for several health plans. That fact, however, did not seem to be helping them get new patients from the health plans. She asked, "How can we get the word out that we are available?" Word-of-mouth marketing is the most natural way to spread the word.

A regional sales manager for a health plan telephoned to tell me that during the previous few months 90 percent of the new health plan members who were assigned to one medical group had disenrolled from the medical group and the health plan almost immediately. "The problem," he said, "is that we cannot persuade these new members to sign up with another doctor group. They are so angry now, they refuse anything I suggest." Here is an example of how important it is to stop negative word-of-mouth from ruining a practice.

A doctor stopped me in the hallway of a hospital and complained about the slow turnaround time on authorizations. He said, "I have this patient who needs a cardiac stress test. It has been three weeks since I sent in my authorization request form, and I still have no answer. The management of the IPA doesn't return my calls. I'm getting nowhere and am ready to tell all my patients to pull out of the health plans served by that IPA and help them get into the health plans another IPA serves. Then I'll terminate my contract with that IPA. That's the only way I have leverage."

WHY USE WORD-OF-MOUTH IN MANAGED CARE?

I could tell more stories, but these are sufficient to get across the point that even in managed care settings, word-of-mouth marketing is important. In my opinion it is even more important than it is in traditional practices for the following reasons:

1. The stakes are higher. If you mess up in a managed care environment, you can find yourself missing not only a few unhappy patients but a whole group of patients if your contract is terminated.

2. It may seem that patients have less of a choice about their doctor in managed care, but don't fool yourself. Patients still talk about the doctor, the managed care medical group, and the health plan. The word gets around which groups to avoid and which groups to join up with.

3. Many health plans are creating more freedom of choice for their members. If you are under contract with a health plan, it doesn't mean that you will automatically receive referrals from a management office somewhere. New health plan members see your name listed in the provider directory. They will still ask for someone's opinion before coming to your office.

4. Managed care systems have already squeezed the reimbursement rates for physicians. Now, along with pressures from local jurisdictions and the Federal government, they are exerting pressure for improved quality. Patient satisfaction measurements are being taking regularly by health plans and some of the larger multispecialty medical groups. Clinical outcomes are also being monitored as a way to improve quality, weed out undesirable providers, and improve a health plan's marketing capability.

5. Prospective health plan members may select a plan on the basis of their affiliation with the medical group of choice or their hospital affiliation. This sets up a three-way link of incentives to promote member satisfaction. In the past achieving patient satisfaction was looked upon as a matter of "every organization for itself." Now, however, providers who succeed are those who are able to network their patient satisfaction efforts with those of other providers.

6. In some metropolitan areas, competition between health plans and medical groups is so strong that service reputation is the most effective way to stand out from the competition. Low premium or reimbursement prices are not enough. Efficient systems to treat patients and handle information are not enough. Successful organizations refine their systems to promote positive clinical outcomes and measurable patient satisfaction.

7. When employer groups evaluate which health plans and medical groups to recommend to their employees, reputation, as developed by outcomes and patient satisfaction levels, is one of the most important elements in the purchase decision.

WHY MANAGED CARE?

Doctors who decide to get involved with managed care find that this decision brings additional things to think about besides patient care. There are contract issues, utilization review issues, quality improvement issues, capitation, shared risk pools, grievance procedures, and practice guidelines. Once you get used to the new routines, however, you will most likely settle down into a satisfying role as a medical care giver.

Participation in managed care offers a way to revitalize a medical practice. It offers a way to survive in business by maintaining your market share. Managed care offers access to new patient populations. Participating in managed care represents a new way to maintain control over the future.

Clearly, a large group practice with a large proportion of patients in managed care is not for everyone. There will always be a need for private practitioners in solo practices that maintain a fee-for-service patient base. In metropolitan areas, however, the pressures to participate in groups will become enormous. If you feel you are giving up too much control to the health plan or to utilization managers, managed care in the setting of a large group may not be for you. No matter what you decide, word-of-mouth marketing must remain a key part of your overall marketing strategy.

SOURCES OF SATISFACTION AND DISSATISFACTION

Health maintenance organizations offer their members relative freedom from paperwork. Patients know before every visit exactly how much they are expected to pay. This financial stability is appealing. In addition, many health plan members find that they like the physicians in the group. They are competent doctors and have good interpersonal skills.

While there are many benefits to being in a managed care plan, there are also several areas which have caused patient dissatisfaction. In managed care plans patients have less of a choice about their personal doctors. They sometimes feel that they receive only superficial care compared with what they remember receiving under the traditional fee-for-service system. They complain about having to wait for care. If they are out of town, they have difficulty obtaining appropriate care. Members of managed care plans also have more anxiety about the quality of care. Whether these complaints reflect reality is not the point; they do reflect patients' perception, and that is reality.

I've heard the following patient complaints about managed care organizations:

"Why do I have to keep filling out the same forms over and over? Don't they already have this information?"

"I called and was put on hold for ten minutes before someone helped me. By then I forgot what I had called to say."

"My doctor used to be so nice, but since he signed up with that medical group or whatever it is, he acts like he doesn't have the time of day for me."

"I was waiting in the office and they kept letting other people in ahead of me. I waited over an hour while these other people kept coming in and out."

The point is these are sources of negative word-of-mouth and should be dealt with accordingly.

CHALLENGES FOR WORD-OF-MOUTH MARKETING

Developing a consistent word-of-mouth marketing program is challenging for a small private practice, but think about what it means for a managed care group. If you are involved with managed care, you can see the benefits of improved efficiency. The medical group structure you are in offers many ways to save money. Scheduling systems maximize your time, and employees have specialized job descriptions that help them do their work better. What could be better?

Look at it from the patient's point of view. The new structure of the medical group is confusing. The scheduling process has so many policies and procedures to follow that the patient feels that he or she is a burden. What about division of labor? It usually comes across to the patient that no one knows what is going on in the organization as a whole. Larger medical groups have large buildings where patients can get lost on their way to an appointment. There are more departments to watch for, more people to introduce oneself to, more nameless faces who look at a piece of paper in a folder and simply say, "Come in here."

Multispecialty medical groups are the most at risk for negative word-of-mouth. There are many more people who have contact with the patient. This means many opportunities to demonstrate good service but it also means a higher probability that the quality of service will break down at one or more points in the system. The more people who are involved, the higher the chances that the quality of service will vary from one patient to the next.

Large medical groups make the patient feel that there is less of an opportunity to customize the professional-patient relationship, something patients wish had remained from the days of fee-for-service medicine. Then there is this thing which goes on in some back room somewhere called utilization management. To the patient, just call a utilization management committee meeting and it is as if the computer had just shut down and nothing can get accomplished.

In the past it was relatively easy to find one's way around a doctor's office. There was the waiting (a better name is "reception") room, the front office, the hallway leading to the exam rooms, a back office or laboratory, an x-ray room or special procedure room, and a rest room. Walk into a large medical group and it is like walking into a maze. The signs are unfamiliar, there are dozens of doors one is not supposed to use, and the rest rooms are on the other side of the building somewhere on the third floor.

What can be done to enhance word-of-mouth in such a complex setting? Here are some practical things to do to make life easier for managed care patients and promote positive word-of-mouth.

TACTICS FOR SOLO PRACTITIONERS AND SMALL GROUPS

1. Do something unusual for new managed care patients. They come to you with anxieties about quality, access, and service. They know what it was like with a family doctor, and now they have to come to your office. Call them before they enter the office to wel-

come and reassure them. Call them after they leave the office. This phone call can be a short conversation reassuring them that if they have any questions at all, they can feel free to call you at any time. Let them know about any special education programs you have available. Get to know a little about where they work and the type of work they do. In short, show a little interest.

2. One of your loyal champion patients calls you to let you know he or she has to change doctors because the health plan at work requires it. Don't merely say, "Thank you for telling us. We're sorry to see you go," and then hang up. The fact that the patient is telling you about the impending change is significant. A quick thank you will seem like a brush-off, as if you were upset with them for changing health plans. Take the opportunity to celebrate the role they have played in your practice. The longer a person has been a patient, the more important the change is for you and for the patient. Acknowledge it. Celebrate the patient. Have several people talk with the patient on the telephone. Invite the patient into the office for a special going away party which you schedule right in with the rest of your routines of the day. When the patient comes in, be ready with a small gift such as a miniature cake or some other goodie. Tell the patient personally how much you have valued his or her support of the practice over the years and that your reputation is your most important asset. Make the thank you party visible to other patients in the office. Make it short and to the point and send the patient off with hugs and warm smiles. You will benefit from such a positive action.

3. Print a list of health plans you are contracted with and give the list to your champion patients. Tell them "Sometimes people sign up with a new health plan and don't know which doctor to choose. Feel free to let your friends know that we are a provider with their health plan and are welcoming new patients." Post the same list at the front desk or in the reception room for patients to see when they check in for appointments.

4. Work directly with employer groups to get more referrals from the Preferred Provider Organization (PPO) you have signed up with. The more visible you become at the factory or warehouse, the more likely it is that employees will see your name pop out at them when they

read the health plan's provider list. When you go to the work site, make sure to tell at least one or two people you are a provider listed in the provider book. Here are a few ways to create word-of-mouth at these companies:

a. Conduct a free health screening event.
b. Offer complementary physical exams to a few line supervisors.
c. Write a regular health column in the inhouse employee newsletter.
d. Team up with a specialist and give a series of lunchtime lectures on occupational health topics.
e. Place in your waiting room a special notebook with the company's name prominently on the cover. The notebook contains thank you notes from employees and staff of the company who are satisfied patients.
f. Sponsor a table at the annual company barbecue.
g. Join the service club that the company president belongs to and develop a friendship.
h. Make a list of all current patients who work for that company and send them a letter about the things you are doing with the company.
i. Ask some of the champion patients who work for this company how you can spread the word that you accept their insurance (let them suggest some tactics).

TACTICS FOR HMOs, IPAs, AND MEDICAL GROUPS

1. New health plan members represent the most important opportunity to create a positive first impression. Make it a practice to call each new health plan member to let that person know you are glad he or she is are part of your group. Inform the patient that he or she is welcome to come to the office anytime for a free checkup or physical exam covered by the health plan benefits. The sooner you can get such a patient into the office for a positive experience, the

sooner that patient can become a champion for you and the sooner that patient's anxiety will dissipate. It will take a lot of time for someone to make all those telephone calls, but it is worth the investment to set the champions on their way to talking about how great your organization is. Why wait to have champions speaking positively about you to others?

2. Educate, educate, educate. Send a benefit summary to all new plan members enrolled in your group, highlighting the free preventive services they have coming to them. Give them a series of short descriptions of things such as procedures for choosing a physician, how to use the health plan grievance procedures, how to get a referral to a specialist, and where to get emergency care. Assume that each person in the plan is new to managed care. They don't understand all the abbreviations you use (HMO, PPO, IPA, UR, TQI, to name a few). They don't know how things work behind the scenes. If your champion patients understand the behind-the-scenes work, they will have a lot to say to prospective members. They compare what they get from your organization with what they remember getting when they had a fee-for-service relationship with a doctor. Educate them about the benefits of your system. Video cassette and audio cassette versions of these educational materials should be available for those who want to hear and see the answers to their questions. Create a video tour of your facilities to orient new members on where to go for care. These videos can be shared with their friends and families.

3. When a new plan member comes in for a visit, include a five-minute tour of the office that includes meeting the key people. If you are in a large building with several floors of medical services, extend the tour to other floors and give a guided tour from the elevator telling health plan members what is on each floor. If other people are riding the elevator, there is nothing wrong with having them hear where things are located. If there are two or three new members in the office at the same time, have them join the tour. It is best if someone from member services or patient services gives the tour since it is the tour guide with whom the patients tend to bond first.

4. Monitor your disenrollment rate regularly. Make follow-up telephone calls to all the persons who bail out of the relationship to find

out why they are dissatisfied. Communicate the results of this research to both marketing and administration. If you find that there is dissatisfaction with another provider, contact the administration and patient services departments of that organization to let them know how important this is to you. Follow up the telephone call with a letter summarizing the disenrollment event.

5. Your member relations department exists for more than just solving problems after they come up. Member relations promote word-of-mouth marketing for the whole organization. This department's important tasks include the following:

a. The department must identify champion patients and other opinion leaders who can improve your reputation. Make written list of people who are champions. The member relations director should have a weekly or biweekly meeting with the marketing and planning departments to compare information about specific members who are thought to be opinion leaders. During this meeting innovative ideas can be created for managing the relationship between the organization and its champions. To assist them in their work, member relations representatives should interview patients on a regular basis to check on service quality and look for indicators of champion patients. If marketing identifies members who have referred others to the practice, both marketing and member relations can get involved in acknowledging this. Coordinating their appreciation will prevent their stumbling over each other in an effort to show gratitude to champions.

b. Once champions have been identified, member relations must communicate with these individuals on a regular basis in person, on the telephone, and through the mail. The logical starting point is for member relations to call champion patients, introduce themselves, and check to see how the patients are finding the services. Representatives can also give the names of champions to key people in the organization such as receptionists, schedulers, office nurses, and physicians.

c. Member relations should be given the responsibility for advising the administration about any matter which may be causing patient irritation or frustration. Here the team is constantly on the lookout for problems before they come up. In large complex organizations, the key areas to watch are registration, scheduling, reporting, patient education, and relationships with outside organizations to which patients may be sent for services.

d. In managed care organizations there is typically a contractual relationship between your group and other providers, such as hospitals, home health care companies, and skilled nursing facilities. When your patients or their family members experience irritations or frustrations with these organizations, this reflects directly on you. Constant feedback (in person and in writing) should be given these to providers to keep them informed about problems. Here member relations will work closely with the contracting department in communicating with outside providers. When problems do come up, it is vital to coordinate your problem-solving work closely so that the patient is not overwhelmed with calls from a variety of organizations. This can be confusing and frustrating to the patient. Ideally, one person should maintain immediate contact with the patient. This person's job is to coordinate the solution and communicate that solution to the patient before, during, and after the process.

e. Education and training are needed to keep other departments aware of the importance of positive experiences for patients. Member relations can serve as the educational coordinator for this continuous process. Specific examples of how patients are cared for in your organization should be used as often as possible to emphasize the skills needed to enhance your ability to serve.

f. Solving problems immediately for any patient is the task which member relations staff members put at the top of their work lists whenever these situations come up. Here the most important principles are speed, constant communication with the patient, close follow-up with staff members who are assigned the responsibility for clearing up problems, and confirming several days and weeks later that the problem was solved to the satisfaction of the patient. Always document the details of the problem, how it was solved, and the final outcome in the mind of the patient. Monthly meetings with the administration should include a summary of these service opportunities along with documented evidence that similar problems will be prevented in the future.

6.   Consider adding extra amenities such as a toll-free telephone line, no-hassle paperwork which is taken care of for members, telephones to arrange for transportation or check on children, transportation to and from the office, a flower delivered to each patient admitted to the hospital for an overnight stay, and instant customer service anywhere in the organization no matter who the member talks to.

7. Give members more information about the doctors and other providers you work with. An ideal (but expensive) way to deliver this type of information is to produce a series of short video talk shows featuring key physicians being interviewed by a host. At a minimum, make available short resumes on the physicians, in the reception areas or through the mail, to patients who are making a first-time visit to one of these doctors.

8. IPAs and medical groups should consider the health plan as a consumer and create a first impression that overwhelms them with positive feelings. Assign a person to act as the liaison with your health plans to make sure operations go smoothly. The start-up time with any contract is crucial in the process of working out solutions to unforseen problems. If you maintain constant communication between your staff and the key people in the health plan, you will create an atmosphere of trust that will build your reputation. Some areas that can experience snags include the following:

   a. Credentialing of the doctors with a health plan
   b. Orientation to each other's procedural requirements
   c. Processing claims
   d. Scheduling
   e. Utilization review and quality improvement
   f. Reporting

Chapter 10

Breaking Through Cultural Barriers with Word-of-Mouth Marketing

The most significant cross-cultural challenge you face as a healthcare provider involves your assumptions about patients from other cultures. Whenever a patient comes in speaking a different language; dressed in unusual clothing; holding a different set of beliefs about life, health and doctors; having an appetite for unusual foods; and evaluating social classes differently, you will be faced with this challenge.

These cultural traits make us what we are regardless of our heritage or the color of our skin. Frequently, the cultural traits of patients conflict with modern medicine. When this happens, extra care is needed to prevent negative word-of-mouth and promote positive reports about your office.

When the first representatives of a cultural group moved into your area, they had no choice but to get healthcare from folk healers and, when they failed to help, from doctors who practiced American-style medicine. Reports of their experiences spread to others coming into town. Doctors who were careful to respect the cultural traits of their ethnic patients benefited from positive word-of-mouth, while less culturally sensitive doctors suffered from negative word-of-mouth. This is not unique to the healthcare industry; it is the same for almost all businesses.

Word-of-mouth reports are stronger than advertising within ethnic groups. In many cases, paid advertising totally falls flat because of the negative word-of-mouth: too many stories have been told that create distrust and hesitation. What should be a response-getting communication piece results in no response from the cultural groups because of negative word-of-mouth or because the advertising is out of touch with cultural dynamics among those maintaining their ethnic identity. Can you overcome this with more advertising? No. Can you solve it with culturally sensitive advertising? Maybe, but this isn't the total answer since word-of-mouth is the primary source of credible information within ethnic groups.

CULTURE'S POWER

In North America, two forces are at work molding culture. The dominant culture, which already is a melting pot, encourages minority groups to blend into the American way of life. This influence is willingly accepted because many people in ethnic and cultural subgroups want to share the American culture. As they borrow from American culture, their lives change and they become integrated with what they see around them. The other force is the drive to maintain cultural identity. Ethnic heritage is powerful enough to maintain dietary habits, personal hygiene habits, core beliefs about health and healers, and family activities. When a patient comes into the office, you don't know immediately whether that patient is open to cultural assimilation or wants to maintain his or her cultural identity. It is a risk to assume the former.

If, however, the patient is trying to hang on to his or her cultural identity in an illness situation, you could be setting yourself up for negative word-of-mouth unless you approach the situation carefully and gently. Sometimes the patient seems happy with the American style of medicine but a family member is offended because the patient did not follow culturally accepted behaviors for getting well. Or maybe the patient will be are accused of using the wrong doctor. You may become the target of this type of anger. In that case, you will be challenged to remain calm, stepping back emotionally to view what is going on.

CULTURE IS LEARNED BEHAVIOR

Culture has power in our lives because we learn cultural and ethnic ways of behaving from infancy. We learn that some foods are acceptable and some are not. We learn that certain symbolic and some practical tools and materials are needed in the household to carry on the normal routines of life. We learn the language of the family as well as its beliefs about how things should be.

Culture is taught to us explicitly by our significant family members and social leaders. It is taught implicitly by modeling behavior in our presence so that there will be no mistakes. Culture is also powerful because it is an integrated way of living and thinking. Ethnic identity is not merely a collection of things to eat, wear, do, and say. It involves the internalizing of these things as well as what they mean to us. Because of culture's power, it is often easier for a physician to learn the existing cultural expectations and attempt to work within those guidelines than to try to force all patients to "do it our way or else."

People from all cultures also learn culturally accepted health and illness behaviors. They learn to give explanations for their illnesses. For example, in some cultures illness may be seen as resulting from shameful behavior or of supernatural forces that are out of a patient's control. Your patients may have a well-developed list of medical labels which describe their illnesses, but do not assume that they mean the same as what you mean by the same label. The meaning of the symptoms is as important as knowing the cause of the disease. Do your patients, for example, believe that if the symptoms go away, the disease is gone too? Do they fear the treatment as much as the disease and thus withhold information or avoid coming to you until the situation becomes serious? Do they try to use self-care or go to see a folk healer first? The answer to any of these questions may be yes. It depends on the patients and their background.

108 Patients Build Your Practice

COMMON VALUES BUILD YOUR REPUTATION

Fortunately, some common values cross cultural lines and span generation gaps. In general, people from all cultures value hospitality, though it may be practiced slightly different in one culture than it is in another. All cultures value giving and generosity, defined in their own terms. All cultures value obedience, learning, peacemaking, and reciprocity. Use these common threads as links with your patients from ethnic groups other than your own. In other words, if you are not sure what to do in a situation, be sure to include healthy doses of hospitality, reciprocity, generosity, and giving. If you do this, your positive reputation will precede you.

WHAT TO WATCH FOR

If you practice medicine in a metropolitan area, you know that pockets of ethnic subgroups are clustered in neighborhoods. Drive the main business streets and you can see the cultural influences of shop owners reaching out to their constituents. If you are not sure what the ethnic mix of your city is, contact the local library and ask to see the most recent reports from the U.S. Bureau of the Census. In these reports you will be able to identify specific neighborhoods that have the highest concentrations of various cultural groups.

People from some ethnic groups sometimes prefer a less formal environment for healthcare and a practice that appeals culturally to them. They highly respect doctors and their training but can be intimidated or even offended by the formal language and activities in a doctor's office. What you think of as professionalism may be seen as indifference. If you give them a long list of medical advice, they may feel put down. When they develop trust in a doctor, however, they are very loyal, working hard to tell other people about the doctor. Their compliance will be greater also.

The close family ties between ethnic patients create a natural grapevine for your reputation. After a patient visits you (such patients usually prefer treatment in an office rather than in the hospital), the whole family may get together to discuss the event. Besides the illness and the symptoms, you and your work are central to the discussion; this is word-of-mouth marketing at its best.

Women are the guardians of health in many ethnic communities. Older women and women with experience caring for sick family members are seen as holding important wisdom. They can also be a good referral source since they understand their own limitations when it comes to curing disease.

IDENTIFYING THE OPINION LEADERS

The constant challenge in word-of-mouth marketing is identifying the opinion leaders. This is especially true when a doctor is attempting to build a reputation within an ethnic subculture. Here are some suggestions to help you in this process.

There are two types of cultural opinion leaders to focus on. Some people are the cultural innovators, the ones who are trying to assimilate into the dominant culture. These people maintain a close connection with their social roots but also go outside their own groups to explore American culture. They tend to be better educated and have had more exposure to American medicine. The greater the distance between themselves and their relatives who have immigrated, the more they will follow American medical culture. They travel out of their neighborhoods and listen to communications from the American culture. Most of these individuals are found in metropolitan areas, where they can experience the full range of American culture. They take classes in local colleges to improve their ability to interact with the American culture. These cultural risk takers are followers of American culture. The people they have contact with in the mainstream culture are their opinion leaders. For many people, these opinion leaders represent what it means to be successful.

Those who follow the lead of cultural innovators also want to assimilate into the larger culture. They aspire to become successful and intentionally imitate the innovators. They accomplish this through repeated personal communication with innovators, by observing their behavior, and by reading about the experiences of innovators and the results they achieve. This information encourages them to continue the quest and cautions them to avoid the problems others have encountered.

The other opinion leaders are the cultural traditionalists who are looking to maintain their cultural forms. They wish the innovators would use old styles of healing and medicine that incorporate the deep spiritual dynamics of the community. Traditionalists may view innovators as prime examples of what to avoid. These individuals prefer speaking their own languages and sometimes refuse to use English even if they can speak it. They are less likely to experiment with external cultural traits such as food, clothing, and entertainment. They may prefer to stay at home rather than go into what is perceived as a hostile environment. They highly regard cultural self-sufficiency and have strict codes of discipline.

When it comes to healthcare, many cultural traditionalists are forced to come to American doctors simply because there are not enough physicians in their own groups. When they come to your office, they are afraid that you will ask them to do things which go against their beliefs. They are afraid that you will not understand them. They are concerned that they will not understand what they have to do to receive care. What can you do to address these feelings and at the same time build your reputation? Here are a few suggestions:

1. Hire employees who are bilingual. This is especially important in metropolitan areas where dozens of cultural subgroups live. Employees who speak the appropriate language can soothe patients' fears and anxiety. They can also be an ally in building confidence in your skill. Avoid using children to translate. When you do use a family translator, ask the person to translate word for word without interpretation. Also ask that person to seek clarification if there is any doubt about anything you say. If you do not have a bilingual staff, contact representatives of the cultural groups you serve and tell them you are looking for volunteers to help with translation. Explain why you need translators: you want to minimize anxiety and fear and promote trust in the healing process. Sign up the volunteers on a roster and establish a telephone alert protocol. By asking patients at the time of

scheduling or at the time of the first visit if they need a translator, you can help the volunteer team plan ahead. Tapping into a volunteer pool will start a round of positive word-of-mouth which will probably result in more patients. Make sure to find ways to acknowledge and show appreciation to these volunteer translators.

2. Evaluate the level of assimilation into the American medical culture before you go too far with the diagnosis and treatment. In the initial interview, assess the American education level, previous experiences with American medical providers, family immigration history (illegal aliens may decline to tell you the truth for fear of exposure), and whether their American experience is urban or rural (urban immigrants tend to be more sophisticated in using medical services).

3. Ask what the women think about the illness. The answer to this will give you valuable clues about what the illness means, how they think they got the disease, and what they think will help cure it. If the patient mentions the name of someone you think may be seen as a folk healer, ask for permission to meet that person. This can only help build your credibility.

4. Actively cultivate a relationship with local folk healers. They can be one of your best referral sources if you have their trust. They also can block referrals and counteract your medical advice if they distrust you. The best way to identify them is to get to know some of the families in the area. As trust develops between you and these families, you will be able to ask who they turn to for health advice. Once you have identified the ones with health wisdom, make a point to get to know them personally. They are interested in doctors because people turn to them all the time for medical advice. If you are friendly and do not rush the relationship, they will like you, and this will begin translating into referrals. In turn, you can do them a favor by giving them up-to-date information about scientifically accepted treatments.

5. When you develop a list of ten to fifteen folk healers, invite them to a free medical seminar that you will host. You are the featured speaker at this event where you give them practical information on how to recognize difficult cases and when to refer to a trained physician. Teach them a few practical things they can pass on to the

people who depend on them for medical wisdom and then be prepared for the referrals that will start coming your way.

6. <u>Give free care to these folk healers to develop referral bonds</u>. Show them extra attention when they come into the office for a complimentary visit. Be careful, however, not to give them large amounts of free sample medications as you cannot control their distribution of these medications.

7. <u>Study the communication style of folk healers</u>. As you incorporate some of their interpersonal skills in your work, you will build your reputation. Practice talking about the meaning of illness with your patients.

8. <u>If older members of the cultural group receive extra respect, give the same to your older patients</u>. Practice politeness and warmth.

9. <u>Incorporate ethnic alternatives into your nutritional recommendations</u>. If you are unsure what you can prescribe that is culturally acceptable, take a nutritional history and have it interpreted by someone from the group. Then make recommendations based on the patient's usual fare.

10. <u>Make sure to spend time with ethnic patients</u>. They look up to you and respect your training. They want to hear about their illnesses directly from you. They expect to hear answers to their unspoken anxieties regarding severity, prognosis, seriousness of symptoms, and the rationale for your prescription. If you give this to your nurse to do, these patients will leave disappointed, believing you are incompetent.

11. <u>Check your assumptions about the cultural groups represented among your patient records</u>. You are at risk if you make generalizations about all people in an ethnic group based on the behavior of just a few.

12. <u>Remember that there are individual differences between people within a cultural subgroup</u>. If the other suggestions aren't enough to keep you alert, this one will.

13. <u>Patients from some ethnic groups will probably perceive greater risk in trying a new doctor for the first time</u>. If you give them a little extra time during the first few visits, you will minimize their anxiety

and build your credibility. Instruct your staff members on this point. Help them remember that if you rush the care, you will leave these patients confused, disappointed, and fearful, setting yourself up for negative word-of-mouth.

14. Some people from other cultures see more value in the tangible evidence of your credentials. Placing your diplomas and certifications prominently in the office will add to their trust in you. If you have published articles in medical journals, make a bulletin board display of the first page of each article. If you give lectures at a medical school, hospital residency, local college, or community group, put up copies of announcements or programs that list the topics of your speeches. These can be silent reminders that you have the skill to care for their needs.

15. Be aware of the pride people have in their heritage. Attend parades and festivals to discover the important cultural traits. If you attend the annual parade, for example, bring some artifacts and decorations to the office which remind people of this event. When ethnic patients come into the office before and after the event, make sure to talk about the holiday with them, wishing them good luck and good health as they leave the office.

16. Be careful in using American idioms. Someone learning the English language can easily be confused by many commonly used American phrases. Listen to yourself talk, and if you use an idiom, define it to make sure you have not made it more difficult for the patient to understand you.

17. Don't assume that your self-care recommendations will meet with wholehearted acceptance. Even if the patient nods his or her head about something you direct them to do, do not assume that the patient is agreeing with you. The patient may be trying to be polite when the probability of actual compliance is remote.

18. Educate yourself about cultural taboos to avoid in the office and in self-care follow-up education. People from some cultures are offended if they are touched on the head, have to show the bottoms of their feet, or are asked to change their diet. Your best chance of learning is to get to know a champion patient's family. Invite them to

your home to eat a few times. As the two of you feel more relaxed, you will be able to ask questions about idiosyncracies you should be aware of. Ask before trust is built, however, and you will not get an answer. The fact that you are genuinely interested in their culture will get around the grapevine quickly. The fact that you invited a champion patient to your house for dinner a few times or went to the patient's house to eat will also become part of the positive reputation you are building.

19. Incorporate culturally accepted home remedies into your prescriptions. This builds on what they already believe to be true. If you explain why some of their favorite home remedies actually work, they will talk about your knowledge to their friends and families.

20. Translate your signs, instructions, and forms into appropriate languages. This will make the office more accessible.

21. Train the office staff in the differences between cultures on points such as the following: meaning of symptoms, expectations of physicians' and nurses' behaviors, perceptions about the severity of illnesses, beliefs about doctors, and perceptions about how vulnerable the patient feels.

22. Allow patients to include their entire family in the diagnosis and treatment process. If the patient hesitates in making a commitment to follow medical advice, it could mean they want to discuss the matter with their family first.

Chapter 11

Word-of-Mouth Marketing for other Specific Groups

I have emphasized the importance of developing strong relationships with champion patients and referral sources. Now I'm going to ask you to take those principles one step further and use the power of networking in community groups with the help of your champion patients. Although this chapter focuses on networking with organized groups, all your word-of-mouth marketing should be seen as a form of networking.

Every community has a network of powerful communication grapevines. These channels of energy are used to do more than pass gossip; they are a popular means of getting things done. If you want to have a strong ally in building your reputation, tap into the community grapevine. Opinion leaders often give, withhold, distort, clarify, confirm, evaluate, and edit information about people and events. If the right person gets positive information about you, the news will travel like a grass fire in a windstorm. Negative news travels even faster.

Your public relations task is to link in with both the formal and informal connections your patients have with other people in the community, many of whom fit the champion profile. However, many practitioners fail to create a synergy between the rest of their reputation-building work and public relations with community groups. It is as if the two were totally unrelated when in fact they are brother and sister.

Here are a few examples of community groups to look for.

1. One type of group consists of the informal friendships between people at a similar stage in life or with similar vocational or avocational interests. A group of young mothers taking turns baby-sitting for each

other, a group of men who go on a quarterly fishing trip, and the friendships between private pilots who fly for relaxation are examples of informal friendships. All represent opportunities for your practice.

2. Another type is the formal membership group that comes together to help its members achieve a common goal. Examples include the local amateur radio club, the philanthropy group at the community hospital, the women's auxiliary of the university, and the downtown business association.

3. An open group is one that is loosely structured and allows people to drift in and out without making a commitment. This is the case with the people who seem to end up together at the local baseball park on summer nights to cheer on the home team and the people who take part in semiannual walkathons and races that benefit a local charity.

4. Other groups are closed because membership is closely controlled. More stable membership exists in closed groups because the people know each other better. Closed groups include organizations such as membership-by-invitation service clubs, the employees from the nearby factory, and the local church's board of directors.

It is not important to precisely categorize each group in the community since many groups fit into more than one category. What is important, however, is to begin looking for opportunities to tap into the power of these groups through your patients and their relationships with group members.

Groups fulfill several needs for patients. For example, They provide a sense of belonging. When patients attend group meetings and get involved in group functions, they focus on the people around them instead on themselves. Group meetings are structured settings for communication with others. Even if formal "group business" is conducted at a group meeting, there is always informal social interaction before, during, and after the meeting. When your patients participate in groups, they have an opportunity to learn and practice new roles modeled by others. They learn what is culturally acceptable and test the limits of acceptability by asking questions, observing behavior, and making comments. Groups help people grow and change. The members of a group have a common purpose or function when they work together. Finally, groups provide a setting in which things can be done together.

Group communication affects everyone in the group. When patients attend group meetings, their attitudes are shaped unconsciously. They develop enduring values and specific opinions about a variety of issues,including healthcare. There is so much power in group communications that sometimes group members or their friends will act on a suggestion because of where it came from rather than critically evaluating its content. A few high-visibility leaders in a group can, through their charismatic way with people, sway opinions on a variety of subjects, including healthcare and healthcare providers.

HOW TO PICK A COMMUNITY GROUP

Almost every book on public relations for healthcare professionals suggests that the doctor get involved with a few social groups in the community. While I don't disagree with this, I recommend that the doctor analyze carefully which groups are the best ones to get involved with. There may be many groups with which you will have brief contact, but you will probably choose to become a member of only a few.

The local library or chamber of commerce has a printed list of the various community groups in the area. As you read the list, think of the types of patients your practice attracts: Are you looking for children, adults with certain chronic diseases, or people in a certain social class? If you are not sure what types of groups your favorite patients belong to, look through your charts and create a profile of the typical patient and patient family. Start asking patients what groups they belong to or what groups they want to belong to. Make a note of the groups in which your patients hold formal or informal membership. Are these the types of groups you or your spouse could join? Are they the types of groups you would be glad to support with your volunteer time, attendance, and donations? Remember that informal groups are usually not listed in official directories.

There are two marketing strategies to choose between when one is thinking about community groups. The first is the strategy of maximizing the contacts you already have because you have happy patients holding membership in these groups. Second, is the strategy of expanding your reach by getting involved with new groups. The champion-type people in those new groups will help you tap the resources of other grapevines. Whatever strategy you select, stay with it for enough time to see whether it is working. Six to nine months is the average minimum time needed to scope out the opportunities and determine whether your networking efforts are paying off.

Your constant challenge in networking is identifying and working with opinion leaders. Because you are a healthcare professional, group leaders are likely to ask your opinions and ideas. They will respect your background and training even if they know nothing about how you treat patients. When this happens, do as the ancient proverb suggests: count others better than yourself. If you do, the group leaders will talk about you to others.

WORKING WITH A VARIETY OF GROUPS

You won't have time to get involved with every type of community group. In addition, you have your own interests to consider. Long-term involvement with a group suggests that you get enjoyment from the process. If you are not a joiner, there are still opportunities to tap the power of word-of-mouth in groups. Here are a few suggestions for working with some of the more common social groups.

1. Women's groups. Women are the leading decisionmakers in healthcare. They are usually the ones who choose to take a sick child to the doctor. Sometimes they make doctor's appointments for the men in their lives. Because of their experience with physicians, women are experts at selecting a new doctor. They know about waiting, scheduling, and paying for healthcare. They know doctor's office staffs. Listen to what they say and you will learn how your reputation can be enhanced.

In each community there are usually several women's groups,

most of which will welcome a doctor speaking on a health issue that is important to them. Contact the local library or university to find out which groups are around. Compare this list with what your female patients tell you about the groups they belong to. Have the office manager or office nurse offer to speak to a women's group on a health topic. Let them suggest who to talk with to make the arrangements or let them talk with the leaders directly. If you involve a champion patient in the process, you will get much more word-of-mouth about that speaking event.

Besides the organized groups they belong to, many women also have informal communication networks which can contribute to your reputation.

2. <u>Employer groups</u>. Many physicians have tapped successfully into the working groups in the community. Lunch-time brown-bag lecture series work in some companies. Helping a company design a wellness program and then giving health education lectures as part of the program builds your reputation.

You can also tap into the power of the corporate grapevine by letting your champion patients speak for you. Make a list of the major companies your patients work for. The office nurse can suggest to champion patients a few ideas about how you can help their companies develop health promotion and disease prevention programs. Ask the champion patients if there is a company newsletter. Ask them how you can communicate to other workers that you accept their type of insurance. Examples include putting up personal notices on the company bulletin board. You can contact businesses yourself but probably will not be allowed to put up a notice that you are accepting new patients. Your champion patients have the clout to get that done for you, so let them try.

3. <u>Hospital nurses and technicians</u>. When I give lectures on word-of-mouth marketing, I suggest that people interested in tapping into the power of the grapevine should start with what is most natural in their line of work. For doctors, the most natural starting place is with nurses. When you have a solid reputation with nurses, move out to the rest of the community. There is no community group more adept

at promoting your reputation than the nurses you see every time you go to a hospital or skilled nursing facility.

Because of my work I get frequent calls asking me to recommend a doctor. Often I am tempted to say, "Go up to the medical-surgical unit and ask the nurses there." That reflects reality. Nurses know physicians better than anyone else knows them. They see doctors at their best and worst. They observe your bedside manner, and they know quickly whether they will recommend you to a friend. Patients ask them for personal recommendations, and believe me, nurses give detailed recommendations based on their own experience or what they have heard through the hospital grapevine.

Once I did a test with a group of hospital nurses to see how easy it was for them to identify physicians to recommend to others. I asked them, "Who would you recommend to someone who needs a doctor?" I was more interested in how they gave a response than in the specific names they came up with. First, in nine of ten cases, the nurse knew without hesitation whom he or she would recommend, blurting out the name almost before the question was completed. Second, they were not content with just giving a doctor's name. They embellished the name with a variety of positive qualifiers and observations about the doctor's behavior. Third, half the nurses volunteered the name of a physician they definitely would not recommend to someone. They said things like "I wouldn't recommend Dr. _____, he" or "I would stay away from Dr. _____, he is"

I realize that this was not a scientific study and that nurses responding to me as a member of the healthcare community talked to me a little differently than they would have talked to a prospective patient. They know how to be discreet. However, they seem to have strong opinions about which doctors to recommend and which ones to avoid. Tap into this conviction. It is a powerful force in word-of-mouth marketing. It reminds me, however, that the single most important action you can take to enhance word-of-mouth marketing is to be congenial toward the nurses you work with. In many ways they can be your greatest supporters and they will send you a lot of patients.

A seminar series just for nurses or allied health technicians that you teach in the hospital will enhance their perception of your competence. Pick topics that are interesting to them or that relate directly to making their work more productive. Keep the seminars short and, above all, practical. Their supervisors and the hospital education department will be glad you are participating in in-service education (the nurses may even get continuing education credits for the time you spend with them). Seminars are a great way for you to get to know these hospital employees better as people. It will change the way you deal with them in the patient care area.

4. <u>Seniors.</u> One of the most important topics of discussion among seniors is personal health. This is the time of life when people are the heaviest users of healthcare services. Seniors know how important health is; they have had to become wise healthcare consumers. Opinion leader seniors are also at the time of life when they can say what they please and let the chips fall where they may. Seniors are often looked up to for advice. For all these reasons, you should tap into the powerful energy of word-of-mouth marketing among seniors.

There are a variety of senior groups, many of which enjoy having a doctor give a speech on a health topic in which they are interested. They enjoy asking questions and getting your opinions on the latest medicines or treatments they hear about on the news. Seniors are quick to relate experiences they have had with their own or the family's personal health. This too is good for your reputation. Someday they will be talking about you to someone else.

Interacting with seniors may seem to take all the patience you can muster. You are in a hurry; they have all the time in the world to spend with you. You don't want to hear about what happened to their daughter-in-law on her recent cruise; they want to tell you about someone important to themselves, someone who could be a prospective patient. Unless you are an orthopedic surgeon, you don't want to hear about all the problems that occurred when they had a hip replaced; they want to check your personal reaction to see what kind of doctor you are. As a word-of-mouth marketing specialist I say, "Yes, you do want to hear about these things. These conversations can be rewarding in themselves and give you a chance to develop relationships with champions."

If you become active in a senior organization, the word will spread like wildfire. "Did you know that Dr. _____ is a member of our group? She is such a nice woman" will be the type of thing they say. They know how busy doctors are and know that few take the time to get involved with seniors groups at the grass-roots level.

As seniors advance in age, their offspring or legal guardians are charged with making more healthcare decisions. It is therefore imperative for you to cultivate relationships with a senior patient's most significant care givers. If a patient's offspring live in another city, ask permission of the patient to contact the children with information about the patient's health status. Upon approval, make a phone call or write a short note. Whether they live in your city or not, encourage adult children to maintain contact with your patient. Give progress reports on treatment outcomes and prognoses. Referral word-of-mouth marketing principles apply as much in their case as they do anywhere else: these people know other people their age who have elderly parents who need healthcare. They talk with these people about the health problems of their parents. They talk about the nice, caring doctor who goes the extra mile without being asked, and your reputation improves.

If a patient has a court-appointed professional guardian, or conservator, create a word-of-mouth marketing program for that individual just as you would for any healthcare professional: Be available, take them to lunch, provide information that helps them recognize when they need you or helps them do their own work better, show gratitude for their referrals, and ask for their help in getting other legal guardians to make referrals to you. Legal guardians get paid each time they take one of their clients to see the doctor, and so they are willing to make a referral. They are legally charged with watching over all matters for their clients and are happy when they can keep the clients healthy. These professionals talk among themselves and compare notes on which healthcare providers to avoid and which ones are the most responsive to their clients' needs.

5. <u>Social and Service clubs</u>. A physician told me that he thought it was a waste of time to go to the local chapter of the international service club in his area: "I attended a few meetings, and I got frus-

trated at all the mindless bull that was going on there. I have better things to do with my time than go to lunches all the time." Not everyone sees the value in actively participating in service clubs or Chambers of Commerce. It has to be something you enjoy or your dissatisfaction will quickly show.

Service clubs have a structured hierarchy of leadership. Respect this hierarchy at all costs as you begin networking. It is acceptable to let the person responsible for planning programs know you are available to speak on one or more topics. If you decide to be innovative with business etiquette, be cautious and be sure to follow the formal and informal rules of that particular group. If you ask your champion patients which groups they belong to, you will have a short list of the key groups with which you should begin networking. The next time a champion patient comes into the office for services, let that patient know you have contemplated joining the same group and want to know what he or she thinks about it. What is involved in membership in the group? Ask these questions only after investigating your options and narrowing the field to the commitments you can keep. Why should you tell a champion patient that you are interested in his or her group? It starts the word-of-mouth marketing within that group immediately.

6. Churches. Personal health has a spiritual dimension. I have seen many churches place special emphasis on health once a month. A local physician or nurse is asked to give a very short (five minutes) presentation on a health issue. This gets the doctor up in front and, as in service clubs, uses the power of the doctor's personality to great advantage. I recommend starting by asking your champion patients which congregations they belong to. Take the list you generate and decide on one or at the most two congregations to get involved with. Offer to conduct a personal health series in church at the weekly meeting. You don't always have to do the talking if you can arrange for other health professionals to speak for you.

Churches, like other service organizations, need donations to pay for their overhead. If you can make a modest donation to a special project at the church, you won't get any patients but you will be building a strong reputation. How much is modest is a judgment call.

More important than the money you donate are your time and experience which can be leveraged by the congregation to advance its goals.

7. <u>Neighborhood associations</u>. If you want to find a group of opinion leaders gathered together in one place, attend a local neighborhood homeowners association. The people who attend are the ones to whom others listen. You may have to endure a lot of political intrigue, but this is one of the best groups to use to tap into the grapevine of word-of-mouth. Offer to work on a subcommittee or help plan the annual barbecue in the park. Personal involvement on a consistent basis is the key to success.

HOW TO IDENTIFY PATIENTS' INVOLVEMENT IN GROUPS

A personal conversation with your patients will often reveal a lot about their links with social groups. Here are some ways to get patients talking about their experiences with groups:

1. Do you belong to any clubs or organizations?

2. What does your group do?

3. Tell me about your group.

4. How long have you been a member? (Newer members are still learning the ropes and are typically farther away from those who hold the most influence.)

5. Do you get involved with helping people in the group?

6. Do you hold an office?

Use only the questions you feel are appropriate. You don't want to interrogate your patient with a bank of personal questions. On your list of champion patients, make notes to remind yourself of group affiliations. Don't trust your memory.

HOW TO NETWORK IN SOCIAL GROUPS

Here are a few suggestions on how to network effectively.

1. Start by making contact with groups your patients belong to. Ask champion patients what groups they belong to. When you attend a group meeting, introduce yourself to the people who appear to be the leaders. Look for the champion patient and say hello. Let him or her introduce you to others he or she considers important. Conduct careful observation in group meetings to determine which people seem to be the focal points of conversation. Who receives the most questions? With whom do people gather before and after the meeting?

2. Make a small donation to the group you intend to stay with. If you give a big gift, people may wonder what your agenda is. Remember that groups understand the importance of reciprocity. If you give something too big, you may only get a symbolic gift in return, something which will not help you build your practice. Avoid making pit stops at groups you have no interest in coming back to unless there is a request by one of your champion patients to speak to the group.

3. Avoid making an ostentatious splash in the group. It is much better to get involved at the pace the group sets for you through its activities. Splashy entrances can smack of commercial interest and raise suspicions about your goals. It is much better to get genuinely involved with group activities and help the members with their problems. What we are after here is building your reputation, not grabbing a few patients. If you help them even though you have nothing to gain by it, they will reciprocate after trust has been built. In any case, this is not something you can force.

4. Come early to and stay late at group meetings. These are the most important times for networking. If you swing in at the last minute and then leave early because you have a procedure to do, you won't get much sympathy from those who are at the meeting and probably won't get much accomplished in terms of marketing. If you are chronically late, you will have little opportunity to acknowledge the champion patients you see there. You will be looked upon as someone not completely involved in the group and may be treated as an outsider

for a long time. It is the social time before and after the meeting when the most important group work occurs. It is also during this time that you can have the greatest impact through personal conversation. Before and after the meeting, you can build bridges for later referrals. Don't expect to get referrals immediately, but do expect to follow up on any promise you make to the people you meet there. If you fail to follow up as they expect, negative word-of-mouth may result. If you must choose between coming late and leaving early, study the group to see where most of the informal networking occurs. If most people let their hair down after the formal session, make sure to stay late. If the social hour seems to occur before the formal meeting, get there early.

5. Respect the chain of command in the group. If you are too aggressive in trying to communicate with those who hold the power in the group, you could be shut out before you even get started. Groups are sensitive about following protocol and the unwritten rules of how things work. Be careful to honor the accepted communication patterns.

6. If you are asked by the group's program planner to give a speech, find out the expectations before you deliver the speech. What type of presentation has been received with the most enthusiasm in the past? How much time are you expected to use? Do many of the members have to go to other meetings after the program? Do they like to have time for questions after the speech? When you have clear expectations, stick to your promises. If the meeting is supposed to end at 1 PM, sit down at 12:55 to let the chairperson wrap things up.

7. If there is a question and answer session after your presentation, keep it short, allowing time afterward for people to ask questions in more privacy.

8. Carry your business cards with you to give to anyone who asks for one. Don't flaunt them, but have them ready.

9. Focus on getting to know a few people rather than flitting from person to person and developing a relationship with no one. If a group leader's personality irritates you, you don't have to become

friends with that person. Getting to know that person, however, will pay off later if he or she is one of the opinion leaders.

CONCLUSION

I'm not suggesting that you get involved with a group just to use it to build your reputation. What I do suggest is this:

1. Be aware of the dynamics at work in your community. Grapevines can help and hurt you. If you invest your time in a few well-chosen groups, it is like putting money in the bank.

2. Unless you are involved with some of these highly effective grapevines, you will be a mystery to the community around you. People will not know very much about you, but they will still make up their own minds about what you are like. This could be bad or good. Why take a chance?

3. If you are able to overwhelm a few champion patients with excellent service, the news of your work will get out. By the time the message gets passed to the third or fourth person down the grapevine, it may be slightly altered, but chances are that it will still be positive. It may even be embellished by well-meaning people who listen to your champion talk and then make the report sound even better to the next person. In the process people are getting to know you whether you like it or not. You are building your business the old-fashioned way, through your reputation.

Chapter 12

Conclusion

The ideas in this book can be summed up in two principles:

1. People talk.

2. Give them something good to say.

As you create a word-of-mouth marketing plan, use these principles as a guide and you will succeed.

After dealing with this subject for several years, I have come to the conclusion that professionals involved in personal services industries have an easier time applying word-of-mouth marketing ideas to their situations. I believe this is so for the following reasons.

1. Professionals engaged in personal services are much more likely to know their customers by name. This is true for professionals such as physicians, dentists, veterinarians, chiropractors, counselors, therapists, psychologists, lawyers, accountants, financial planners, hair stylists, and podiatrists. However, this is also true for many high-ticket-product sales professionals, such as real estate brokers, automobile and truck dealers, and contractors. A major challenge in word-of-mouth marketing is being able to identify champion consumers who willingly talk about your service. For someone who manages a mini-market, it is much more difficult to get to know the customers since their buying behavior is slanted toward quick, low-involvement purchases of convenience. It's not impossible to implement a word-of-mouth marketing program in these industries, just a little more difficult.

2. Because of the high involvement with clients, professionals will have more information about the consumer. This is especially true of physicians and psychologists, who have the most private information about a person. Similarly, the consumer will have, through direct

experience, more information about the key people in the healing professions.

3. In these personal service industries the professional has more time with the consumer than is the case in many convenience businesses. In fact, that is one of the things the consumer wants from of the purchase experience: more time with you. This presents both an opportunity and a threat. In a minimarket the shoppers are not interested in learning a lot about the business, the owner's way with people, and the fact that the owner cares about their patronage. The items they buy are low-risk products, and the transaction experience is so routine that there is little opportunity for either problems or exceptional service. Few consumers will tell their friends what an excellent experience they had purchasing a soft drink at the local minimarket. The exception arises when a problem for the consumer occurs at a minimarket. This presents the opportunity/threat situation, for it is at this point that the consumer gets more involved with the business. How the business manager handles the problem situation determines how word-of-mouth marketing is played out. By contrast, medical care services allow the patient to have several different types of high-involvement experiences, any of which can be exceptional, terrible, or mediocre.

To the degree that someone in your business has become truly obsessed with word-of-mouth marketing, you will achieve positive results. Clearly, it takes at least one person in the business to become the proponent of word-of-mouth marketing. Without this person to require adherence to these principles, word-of-mouth efforts will gradually degenerate and eventually fall flat. By contrast, with even one leadership person constantly moving the rest of the staff toward excellence in patient satisfaction, the program will succeed.

If you implement a word-of-mouth marketing program and are not getting referrals from your patients, look at this issue, for it is the single largest reason why such programs do not work. For example, if the doctor or another key person is giving lip service to the concept but is not actively involved in supporting word-of-mouth marketing, the program will have limited success and the patients will receive mixed signals from the office. One staff person with a noncooperative attitude toward word-of-mouth marketing can cancel the good efforts of the rest of the staff. Patients will be confused about whether you provide excellent service or poor service. These patients will end up talking more about the negative than about the positive. It is safe to assume that they will eventually come down off the fence of confusion on the side of negative word-of-mouth.

There are other factors which influence how good a response an office receives from word-of-mouth marketing. If you are in a heavily saturated managed care market, for example, the results may be slower in coming since your champion patients may be talking to people who have a health plan which requires them to go elsewhere for care.

Successful word-of-mouth marketing programs succeed if two parallel tracks are followed consistently:

1. Stopping negative word-of-mouth by aggressively seeking out problems and then taking visible actions to solve those problems as quickly as possible

2. Promoting positive word-of-mouth by implementing some of the ideas in this book

Trying to ride on a single track will cause a program to crash. It's that simple.

Consider the worst case. You have implemented a positive word-of-mouth program but have failed to address the issue of patient dissatisfaction. What have you accomplished? You have been able to bring in a few more people who will quickly join the ranks of dissatisfied patients who talk negatively about the practice. You will end up doing more and more to get less and less. Conversely, it is not enough to stop negative word-of-mouth, although this in itself is a commendable achievement. If you don't promote positive word-of-mouth, your problem-solving efforts will be weakened.

Word-of-mouth marketing is

• The most natural way to promote a practice without violating the professional-patient relationship. This is the type of promotion you can do in the normal course of your clinical business. It doesn't require a high-priced marketing consultant to handle the details. I know there are a lot of good ideas here, perhaps too many to implement in one healthcare practice. However, if you pick a few activities you can engage in naturally without disrupting the flow of operations, you will reap rich rewards.

- The lowest-cost promotion method you can find. It also brings the best return on investment of any promotional method I know.

- The lowest-risk promotion program. You risk little cash and a lot of reputation. Every other promotion method requires that you risk heavy doses of both cash and reputation.

- The most powerful form of business development, harnessing the personal communication energy of dozens of people who speak on your behalf and actually bring new patients.

- Highly motivating for employees and patients. When people see that they can get involved and make a difference, they become motivated to do more.

- The most demanding promotional method in that the work is never over. This form of communication requires a commitment, even an obsession, to continuously make it happen. After reading this book, you may decide that this promotion method is not for you. You may decide to spend your hard-earned cash on another promotional method and let someone else handle the details. If you have this attitude, you may be the type of manager who is also letting someone else take care of stopping the negative word-of-mouth. That is a grave mistake in today's marketplace, where consumers are demanding better service and getting it.

- The most enjoyable form of practice management. More than any other management activity, word-of-mouth marketing tactics create a sense of pride, a continual sense of expectancy and hope, and a high degree of involvement for both the staff and the patients.

- The program most consistent with known patient behaviors. People talk.

- The most efficient targeting method known. With word-of-mouth marketing you target specific people who are looking for a doctor. Most other promotional programs are shotgun methods compared with this. Even promotional efforts that focus on narrowly defined population groups miss more than 90 percent of the time.

- The type of promotion most doctors hope for and few plan for.

- Less controllable than some other promotion programs in that you cannot mandate when your champion patients will deliver referral messages to their friends and families. You have ultimate control over direct delivery marketing (what the message is, when it is given, what it looks like and sounds like), but you have to be satisfied with a very low response rate and a lot of wasted dollars. You also have total control over your own personal sales efforts. Yet direct sales in healthcare practices is the highest-cost promotional method.

- Designed for volunteers. Walk down the halls of the local hospital and see all the volunteers working hard to reduce expenses and improve the quality of care. Most healthcare practices do not have an array of volunteers in blue or pink uniforms, but there are a few groups of patients who will gladly volunteer their voices on your behalf. These champions need recruiting (for referrals), training (in what to say about the practice), and rewards just as volunteers do.

Appendix 1

Sample Letters and Forms

Personal letters are one of the best ways to develop a reputation among patients and in the community. It does take time to write creative letters to patients. Personal letters, however, pay off, and over twelve months you will develop a bank of letters to draw from. You will encounter a variety of opportunities to write short, encouraging letters to patients, letters which will be talked about in their families and circles of friends.

Enlist the support of the office staff which can even draft the letters for you. During the year, keep a file of all your personal letters. This file will become invaluable as a time-saver in writing more personal letters. Keep the letters short (one page or less) and to the point. The fact that they received a personal note of any kind from you will be remarkable to your patients.

These are sample letters you can draw from as you communicate with your patients. Revise them as you see fit to meet your specific needs. Remember that the more personal your letters, the more of an impact they will have (see also Appendix 2 for additional ideas about letters you can write).

THANK YOU FOR YOUR REFERRAL LETTER

Dear _____,

Today it gave me great pleasure to serve someone you referred to our office. I know how important it is for the friends and family members of our patients to get encouragement to come to us for their healthcare needs. When someone is looking for a doctor, that person wants to know that the doctor and the staff are competent and that he or she will receive personalized attention. Thank you for your trust in me and our office staff to meet these types of needs when you recommend others to our office. It means a lot to me personally.

If you have any health questions or concerns, please feel free to call me at any time. Also, if there is anything we need to know to improve our ability to serve you, I hope you will be direct in telling me your suggestions. I value your perspective on my work and know that there may be others you will send here for healthcare.

Thank you again for recommending my office. I value your participation in our practice.

Wishing you the best of health,

WELCOME TO OUR PRACTICE LETTER

Dear _____,

Thank you for coming to the office today. I am pleased to have the opportunity to serve your healthcare needs. My goal is to provide you with the kind of competent, personalized attention you need to enhance healing and good health. If you have any questions about the office or about your needs as a result of today's visit, please do not hesitate to call me. I will be glad to speak with you personally.

In the past I have found that many of our patients are recommended to us by their friends or families. I sincerely hope you will find in our office the type of care you would recommend to a friend. If not, I need to know how we can enhance our work for our patients. Please let me know if there is anything we can do to improve our office policies and procedures.

Wishing you good health,

HALL OF FAME INTRODUCTION LETTER

Dear Friends,

You are holding one of the most valuable documents in our office: our Patients' Hall Of Fame book. In this binder are letters which have been sent to us by our patients, thanking us for the care they receive here. Some of the letters have been transcribed for easier reading; the originals are on file in my office.

Each month at our office staff meetings we take a few minutes to celebrate the thank you letters our patients send us. It is a positive way to reinforce high-quality service standards. While these letters say thank you to us, you should know that they have come from patients who have trusted us enough to recommend us to a friend or family member. That is why they appear in this book. Some patients have recommended that just one or two others come here while others have referred many people to us over the years. We truly appreciate their interest in our office and in the competent, personalized care they receive here.

To all of our patients who have thought enough about us to recommend us to friends or family members, we say "thank you".

Sincerely,

WELCOME TO A NEW HEALTH PLAN MEMBER LETTER

Dear _____,

    Welcome to _____ health plan and to the _____ medical group. Since I am one of the primary care physicians in the group, I wanted to invite you in for a complimentary visit to the medical group. I work with a staff of very dedicated professionals interested in providing the best healthcare available anywhere, and I would like to invite you to the office for a personal tour of our facility and introduce you to some of the professionals who will be assisting you when you need medical services. During the tour I will give you written information about our services and how to best use the care we provide.

    Our new member tours are given every Monday evening at 7 PM in our main office at _____ (give address, nearest cross streets, freeway exits needed, etc.). Free parking is available at _____. If you are unable to come at that time, I will make special arrangements for you to come during a time more convenient for you.

    I am honored that you have chosen _____ for your medical services and look forward to meeting you personally.

Yours sincerely,

Appendix 2

Coordinating Word-of-Mouth with Other Promotional Methods

Traditional marketing management is a blend of five elements:

- Patients and their needs
- The mix of services offered
- Access to services
- The cost to the patient
- Promotional/communication methods

Word-of-mouth marketing is a tactic which is ideally suited to managing all these elements, as the following outline illustrates.

1. Patients need information about doctors, reassurance about going to a new doctor the first time, and assistance in decisionmaking. Word-of-mouth marketing fulfills these needs directly and forcefully.

2. Marketing management involves creating the right mix of products and services to meet patients' healthcare needs. The root product or service many physicians offer, however, is competence and communication about health and illness. Word-of-mouth marketing supports these two contributors to successful service by supplying the main topic of discussion when people talk.

3. Access to your services is crucial to getting patients' needs met. If patients find you, get to see you quickly, feel socially accepted, and feel that they can afford your services, they have access. Word-of-mouth marketing helps create access by informing a prospective

patient how to get to you and creating an expectation that they will find acceptance in your practice.

4. In addition to the financial obligation to pay for your services, new patients must overcome their unwillingness to trust you for their healthcare. Word-of-mouth marketing makes it easier for them to give you their trust because they have relied on the word of a person who is satisfied with your service.

5. Communication to current patients, prospective patients, health plans, and other referral sources (including champion patients) is important. Word-of-mouth marketing is the most powerful and cost-effective means of communication. It should guide the overall promotional efforts of your practice.

I have helped many physicians who have tried almost every type of promotional method known in North America. They have tried telephone marketing, direct marketing (through the mail or delivered directly to residences), radio advertising, public relations activities, newspapers, and dozens of other ideas. Some of these promotional ideas work for some doctors but this doesn't mean they will work for you in your community. Some promotional schemes are offensive to both patients and doctors. Many of the traditional methods cost hundreds of dollars before delivering a return. Yet around every corner is someone who promises "results" if you will just buy his or her program.

Let me set the record straight: I have nothing against promotional methods which cost money. I have nothing against advertising or advertising agencies. My point is that if you wish to engage in traditional promotional methods, do so only after reviewing the following considerations.

First, don't advertise at the expense of your word-of-mouth marketing program, the champion patients who are working hard for you already. If you spend all your marketing resources on external advertising and public relations, you will have little left to devote to your champion patients, who are your best marketers. Why take your money out of the bank which gives you the best return and put it in a place where you don't even know the interest rate? Why take the ammunition from the most powerful weapons of marketing in the heat of the battle? Start spending your marketing dollars on your champions: identify them, inform them, encourage them and thank them. Then, if you have marketing money left over, buy a traditional promotional program that is consistent with the reputation you have built.

Second, don't engage in a promotional program that is inconsistent with the best word-of-mouth marketing program you can manage. I've seen medical promotional materials that looked like pizza advertising, but when I went into the doctor's office, the whole atmosphere was different from that of a take-out pizza shop. They had wonderful new patient orientation materials. They were consistent in watching out for small sources of irritation. They treated their champion patients as if the world revolved around them, but their promotional materials were more of a huckster desperate to make a deal with a sucker.

Third, coordinate your word-of-mouth marketing so that its message gets to the right people at the right time. If you are convinced, for example, that direct marketing will get results, for you, you may not wish to give that up altogether. Using this method alone, however, without coordinating it with a word-of-mouth marketing program, is like using only four of the eight cylinders in the promotional engine. Don't ask, "What other promotional methods will we use this year to bring in new patients?" Instead, ask "What additional promotional tactics should we employ that will help us build up word-of-mouth?"

I am convinced that at least 50 percent of the advertising money spent by healthcare practices is wasted because the buyers did not focus the advertising to build word-of-mouth marketing. Instead of informing, encouraging, and rewarding the 20 to 40 percent of patients who are champions, they try to get a 1 or 2 percent response rate from prospective patients with a special offer through high-cost advertising. Many of these patients have a health plan you don't serve. Some will come only for the special offer. Most of the patients who respond to advertising have not had a chance to ask someone else about your practice. They have a high degree of anxiety about their decision to come to you for an appointment. They are unknown to you, as you are to them. It not only costs more to get them in the door, it also costs more to keep them as patients since their anxiety is higher and the risk of losing them is greater. Which would you rather have, the 20 percent who work for you or the 2 percent who may soon abandon you?

OTHER PROMOTIONAL METHODS TO SUPPORT WORD-OF-MOUTH MARKETING

1. Direct marketing and newspaper advertising. If you use direct delivery marketing (that is, delivered by the U.S. Postal Service or a commercial delivery company) to communicate with specific neighborhoods, first determine whether you would feel comfortable sending the material only to your champion patients. Would you be embarrassed if they received this material? Are you uncomfortable about making the same offer to your champions? If the answer to either question is "yes", dump the program and start over.

Direct marketing is the ultimate form of target marketing. You already have the names and addresses of hundreds of patients, the backbone of direct marketing work. If you start with a small list such as your champions, you can control the cost. Direct marketing is my favorite method for a doctor's practice because it confers benefits no other paid promotional effort can match:

a. You control exactly what the patient receives.
b. You control exactly when the patient receives it.
c. You can provide repeat exposures as often as you wish.
d. You can develop a relationship through direct marketing, which you cannot do with other forms of promotion. (For every champion you don't capture through building a productive relationship, you lose the thousands of dollars those champions would have brought in.)
e. You don't have limitations of space and format.
f. Direct marketing can be made personal and confidential.

Direct marketing creates an environment that allows the patient or prospective patient some way to respond, such as coming to the office, calling the office, requesting more information, or telling a friend to come to the office.

I recommend testing a direct marketing program on your champions first. For example, send a series of personal letters to the top fifty or seventy-five champions over six to eight months. Even if it costs something to communicate regularly with your champions, you will be rewarded with referrals many times. Here are some suggested topics:

a. We just redecorated (or remodeled) our office with an award-winning design company. You are invited for a personal tour.

b. The doctor had an article published in a medical journal. We have a summary of it for you, compliments of the doctor.

c. The doctor recently attended a continuing education seminar on the topic of _____. He has made a written summary of the material he presented. We want to share this with you at no charge.

d. We now have a new service available because we just purchased or leased special diagnostic equipment.

e. I will be on vacation in beautiful British Columbia during the month of July. To arrange for a strong continuity of care for your needs, I have made arrangements with Dr. _____ to cover for me when I am enjoying a change of pace. Her phone number is _____.

f. I just returned from vacation and have asked the office staff to put up a display of the pictures we took of our family during our vacation to beautiful British Columbia. Come enjoy this display with us at the office from August 19 through August 26. You won't want to miss the snapshot of my wife and I at . . .

g. We just signed up with a new health plan. If you, a family member, or a friend is signed up with this plan, you may come to our office for care.

h. (From the office nurse) We are holding a special doctor's recognition next week in the office. Can you come? National doctor's day is coming up, and we want our patients to participate by bringing thank you notes to give the doctor.

Please, no gifts other than the thank you notes. We will be placing the notes in a three-ring binder for new patients to see in the reception room. If you want your note included in the notebook anonymously, just mention that at the bottom.

i. The doctor will be speaking at lunch on Wednesday of next week for the Leisure Manor retirement community. He has made special arrangements to invite you to attend even if you are not part of the retirement community.

j. I am happy to hear that you are doing so well after your surgery. It was nice to talk with you on the telephone the other day. Remember to keep following our recommendations.

k. Please accept my sincere appreciation for sending such a thoughtful thank you note. We have a notebook of these kinds of letters we like to share with new patients. May we have the honor of including your letter in the book?

l. Congratulations on your retirement! I know this is a big change for you, and I want you to know that I am available any time you want to discuss your retirement plans. Personal health is more valuable to you now than ever before. Therefore, I am offering you, at no charge, a complimentary physical exam in honor of this occasion.

m. Recently the New England Journal of Medicine published an article on _____, and I wanted you to know about it. The article reaffirms what other researchers have shown: that your diet can be a contributing factor to preventing heart disease. I am enclosing a short summary of the article with this letter. If you would like a complete nutritional assessment, please contact my office. We will be glad to assist you.

n. This week at _____ hospital I gave a lecture on the topic of _____. During the lecture I thought about you and wondered if you would like a summary of the information we discussed. I have taken the liberty of sending it to you. If you have any questions, feel free to contact me at any time. I will be happy to discuss the material with you personally.

o. I recently acquired several copies of a well-known health risk appraisal form which will help you evaluate your health status and your risk of developing various chronic diseases. As a courtesy to you, I am making this short questionnaire available. My office nurse will score the answer sheet and will call you with the results. If you know someone else who may be interested in this health risk appraisal, tell that person to call my office and use your name as a referral.

p.   The office staff is planning a special week honoring the women patients in our practice. We are inviting you to attend our special open house for women on Wednesday afternoon and evening next week between 4 PM and 7:30 PM. My office nurse, Ms. _____, will be showing a short video on health issues. I have also invited a specialist in gynecology to come to our office that afternoon at 5 PM. and make a short presentation on the topic of _____. Please RSVP so we will know how much food to prepare.

Here are a few pointers to boost the effectiveness of direct marketing letters. First, personal direct marketing letters can be long or short depending on the subject covered and what you want to accomplish. Long letters will be read just as much as short ones if you keep the patients' interest, so don't be afraid of long letters. Second, track the results of your direct marketing work. Some letters are just for maintaining a good relationship with patients; others are meant to get someone to take an action. These action-oriented letters require you to count the patients who call or come to the office. Tracking can also mean measuring the dollars you spend on the direct marketing compared with what you collect from those who respond.

A free health screening program is a small perk you can give your champions in exchange for their help in determining whether this program would be well received by others in the community. Leverage the word-of-mouth your champions have going already by letting them bring a friend to be included in the program. Be honest and tell your champions that you are conducting a test to determine whether the health screening is something you should offer on a wider scale. Ask them for feedback on elements of the promotional materials as well as the program itself.

If the program is successful with your champions, encourage them to get involved by recruiting new patients to come to the office. Ask them for the names of people to whom you can send the information, making sure they understand that there is no obligation to become an active patient. This is a good chance for their friends to come in and meet you. If you continue to get positive feedback from your champions, ask them to take information about the offer to the community groups to which they belong. Supply them with small half-page fliers to pass out at meetings they attend. It is acceptable to inform them that you will be spending only a minimal amount on promotion and would like them to help by communicating with people they know. The most important principle here is not to send out a mass mailing or mass delivery for the special program until you have worked your word-of-mouth network.

Before you pay a few thousands of dollars on promotion to unknown neighborhoods to get new patients, hire someone on a project basis to process a series of personal letters from you to each patient (not just the champion patients) who is discharged from the hospital, each patient who has gotten over an illness, each patient who has received positive or encouraging news from a diagnostic test, each patient who sends you a referral, and each patient who is new to the practice. These are just a few ideas. You will be able to think of many more. After you have developed your direct mail program to champions, you can expand it to include the neighborhoods where your patients live. Tell your patients what you are doing so that they can tell their neighbors about it and answer any questions the neighbors may have.

The letters will include reinforcement of the medical advice you gave them, statements of confidence that their quality of life will be improved, and restatements of the benefits of your professional services. Offer to let them call you any time they have a question. Communicate your appreciation for their trust in you and contribution to your reputation. Keep the letters short and personal. If you must use form letters, make sure you read each one you sign to check for consistency with each patient's situation. Don't risk being embarrassed by sending a sympathy letter to a patient who is recovering from surgery. Keep a file of all the letters you send and make notes on the ones which seem to generate the most enthusiasm or the most referrals. When a patient sends a written note in response to your letter, acknowledge that note the next time you see the patient.

2. Exterior signs. Ask your champion patients for their evaluation of the sign on the exterior of your building. Would new patients have difficulty finding the building? Could they spot the sign quickly, or did they have to hunt for it? What exterior landmark is the best reference point for new patients? Would they have a difficult time finding your office in the building? Is the sign easy to read from the car? Is it easy for a new patient to find parking quickly? What would they change to make it easier for other patients to find you? All the information you glean here will be invaluable in helping you get new business: It helps you see reality from your patient's perspective. If you identify problems with your exterior sign, change it to meet the needs of your patients. You can get to your office with your eyes closed, but patients who have never been to the office or who come only once a year see it differently.

3. Yellow Pages advertising. Expenditure for Yellow Pages advertising is on the increase among healthcare practitioners as more and more doctors are deciding to use this promotional method. Graphic artists are developing attractive advertisements for doctors. Your need to purchase display advertising depends on the type of community you are in. Smaller communities may have less of a need for more expensive display advertisements. It also depends on your specialty. If you are a subspecialist, forget Yellow Pages advertising. Instead, spend time building relationships with referring professionals. When you design a Yellow Pages advertisement, make sure it is consistent with your reputation. Do not make glowing promises in the advertisement; this only sets up new patients to be disappointed later. Instead, communicate the facts and benefits clearly and succinctly. Remember that most new patients will depend on the word of at least one other person even if they also see your advertisement.

Appendix 3

Word-of-Mouth Marketing Assessment

INSTRUCTIONS: The following statements describe many offices. Use the following scale to determine how true each statement is for your office. Write a number on each blank line.

1 = very true
2 = somewhat true
3 = not applicable
4 = somewhat untrue
5 = very untrue

_____ 1. No formal, ongoing information gathering process to determine specific areas to improve your service

_____ 2. Do not get specific suggestions or complaints from patients on a regular basis

_____ 3. Some of the office staff consider problem patients as pests or problems to get rid of

_____ 4. Office contact with patients is confusing

_____ 5. Office procedures lack coordination

_____ 6. No acknowledgment/appreciation given to champion patients

_____ 7. Do not know your champion patients are by name

_____ 8. Problem solving for patients is laborious and difficult

_____ 9. Someone at the office undermines positive word-of-mouth or good customer service through indifference or bad attitude

_____ 10. The doctor is not involved in positive word-of-mouth

_____ 11. Get very few referrals from word-of-mouth

_____ 12. Office policies frustrate or anger patients

_____ TOTAL

Score   INTERPRETATION

12–21   Your office is not doing much to build word-of-mouth.

22–31   Your office considers word-of-mouth secondary to other things.

32–41   Your office is about average in implementing a word-of-mouth program.

42–51   With a few improvements, your office will have a strong word-of-mouth program.

52–60   Your word-of-mouth program is probably better than most.

Appendix 4

Medical Group Management Association

The Medical Group Management Association (MGMA) provides comprehensive, timely, relevant resources and valuable networking opportunities for medical practice management professionals in all types and sizes of organizations. MGMA is the oldest and largest professional membership association dedicated to medical practice management. Nearly two-thirds of all physicians involved in group practice in the United States are associated with MGMA member organizations. MGMA understands the wants and needs of practitioners and practice management professionals and is able to provide a broad array of services, products and support to help the medical practice management team achieve positive bottom-line result.

The workplace of MGMA's diverse membership ranges from nationally known clinics to local practices; from freestanding to hospital- and medical school-affiliated medical groups; and encompasses all types of payment mechanisms. In an increasingly complex and competative environment, healthcare marketing takes on added importance across all settings. MGMA is pleased to join with McGraw-Hill Healthcare Management Group in presenting *"Patients Build Your Practice: Word-of-Mouth Marketing For Healthcare Practitioners"*, as a new marketing resource offering many "how to" ideas and action plans.

MGMA provides a variety of services to help meet practice management advocacy, communication, education, information, leadership/professional development, networking and research needs. These services take a variety of forms including publications; an extensive library resource center; workshops and seminars held throughout the country; national, regional and specialty conferences; scholarships; representation in Washington, D.C.; consulting assistance survey and demonstration project reports; professional certification and career planning.

MGMA also offers the expertise and resources of two allied organizations. MGMA's professional certification arm, the American College of Medical Group Administrators, is dedicated to providing certification and networking opportunities for those group practice professionals looking to become the best in the field. MGMA's research arm, the Center for Research in Ambulatory Health Care Administration, is dedicated to providing ongoing research and development in education, new management technology, database services, demonstration projects and valuable survey reports.

EXECUTIVE OFFICE
104 Inverness Terrace East
Englewood, CO 80112–5306
(303) 799–1111
(303) 643–4427 (FAX)

Bibliography

Arnold RM, Lachlin F, Rewarding Medicine: Good Doctors and Good Behavior, *Annals of Internal Medicine*, V.113:10, November 1990.

Bertakis KD, Roter D, Putnam SM, The Relationship of Physician Medical Interview Style to Patient Satisfaction, *The Journal of Family Practice*, V.32:2, 1981.

Crane FG, Lynch JE, Consumer Selection of Physicians and Dentists: An Examination of Choice Criteria and Cure Usage, *Journal of Health Care Marketing*, V.8:3, September 1988.

Dichter H, How Word-of-Mouth Advertising Works, *Harvard Business Review*, V.44, November/December 1966.

Erde EL, Economic Incentives for Ethical and Courteous Behavior in Medicine, *Annals of Internal Medicine*, V.113:10, November 1990.

Glassman M, Glassman N, A Marketing Analysis of Physician Selection and Patient Satisfaction, *Journal of Health Care Marketing*, V.1:4, Fall 1981.

Gochman DS, Stukenborg GJ, Feler A, The Ideal Physician: Implications for Contemporary Hospital Marketing, *Journal of Health Care Marketing*, V.6:2, June 1986.

Hansson RO, Remondet JH, Obrochta D, Bell L, The Dissatisfied Medical Patient: Predictors of Intent to Change Doctors, *Resident & Staff Physician*, V.34:10, September 1988.

Herr PM, Kardes FR, Kim J, Effects of Word of-Mouth and Product-Attribute Information on Persuasion: An Accessibility-Diagnosity Perspective, *Journal of Consumer Research*, V.17, March 1991.

Hill JC, Garner SJ, Factors Influencing Physician Choice, *Hospital & Health Care Services Administration*, V.36:4, Winter 1991.

Kasteller J, Kane RL, Olsen DM, Thetford C, Issues Underlying Prevalence of "Doctor-Shopping" Behavior, *Journal of Health and Social Behavior* V.17, December 1976.

Lauer RH, *Perspectives on Social Change*, Fourth Edition, Allyn and Bacon, Boston, MA, 1991.

Lovelock CH, *Services Marketing*, Prentice-Hall, Inc., Englewood Cliffs, NJ, 1984.

MacStravic RS, Word-of-Mouth Communications in Health Care Marketing, *Health Progress*, October 1985.

Myers JH, Robertson TS, Personality Correlates of Opinion Leadership and Innovative Buyer Behavior, *Journal of Marketing Research*, V.6, May 1969.

Myers JH, Robertson TS, Dimensions of Opinion Leadership, *Journal of Marketing Research*, V.9, February 1972.

O'Shaughnessy J, *Explaining Buyer Behavior*, Oxford University Press, NY, 1992.

Owen C, Formal Complaints Against General Practitioners: A Study of 1000 Cases, *British Journal of General Practice*, V.41, March 1991.

Rogers EM, *Communication of Innovations*, Second Edition, Free Press, NY, 1971.

Ross CK, Frommelt G, Hazelwood L, Chang RW, The Role of Expectations in Patient Satisfaction with Medical Care, *Journal of Health Care Marketing*, V.7:4, December 1987.

Schiffman LG, Kanuk LL, *Consumer Behavior*, Third Edition, Prentice-Hall, Inc., Englewood Cliffs, NJ, 1987.

Schleff T, Shaffer M, How Do Consumers Select Physicians? *Medical Group Management*, May/June 1987.

Shapiro RS, Simpson DE, Lawrence SL, Talsky AM, Sobocinski KA, Schiedermayer DL, A Survey of Sued and Nonsued Physicians and Suing Patients, *Archives of Internal Medicine*, V.149, October 1989.

Smits AJA, Meyboom WA, Mokkink JA, Van Son JA, Van Eijk JV, Medical Versus Behavioral Skills: An Observation Study of 75 General Practitioners, *Family Practice*, V.8:1, 1991.

Stewart DW, Hickson GB, Pechmann C, Koslow S, Altemeier WA, Information Search and Decision Making in the Selection of Family Health Care, *Journal of Health Care Marketing*, V.9:2, June 1989.

Williams SJ, Calnan M, Key Determinants of Consumer Satisfaction With General Practice, *Family Practice*, V.8:3, 1991.

Zaltman G, Duncan R, *Strategies for Planned Change*, John Wiley and Sons, NY, 1977.

Practice Management Titles from McGraw-Hill

Relative Values for Physicians

Baseline Fees for Physician Services

Managing Reimbursement in the '90s

What Are My Fees?

Getting Paid For What You Do

McGraw-Hill OSHA Infection Control Compliance Program

Achieving Profitability With A Medical Office System

The New Practice Handbook

The Personnel Management Handbook

The Complete Medical Marketing Handbook

The Risk Management Handbook

The Clinical Laboratory Management Handbook

Patients Build Your Practice

Medicare Coverage Issues Manual

Medicare Rules and Regulations
(8 Volumes)

HCPCS National Codes and Modifiers

ICD-9-CM, International Classification of
Diseases – 9th Revision

ICD-9-CM Coding for Physicians Offices

CodeLink – Oral & Maxillofacial Surgery

CodeLink – Ophthalmology

CodeLink – Orthopaedics

McGraw-Hill Healthcare Management Group

1221 Avenue of the Americas, New York, NY 10020

1/800/544-8168   Fax: 1/212/512-4138